Follow
To The Best Fruit!

What You Need to Know about Buying, Keeping and Using Fruit

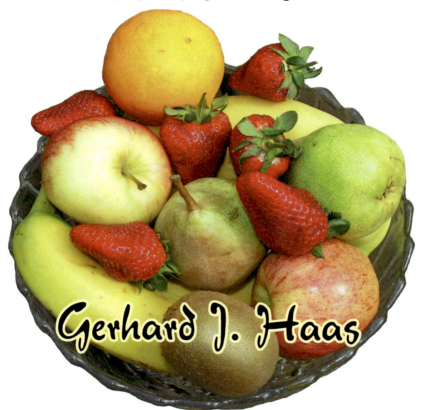

Gerhard J. Haas

Royal Fireworks Press
Unionville, NY

ACKNOWLEDGEMENTS

Many people have helped to bring this book to its present form. The photographs were taken by Dr. Scott Mori, his wife, Carol Gracie, my son David Haas, Irena Yarotsky, Rachel Semlyen and others. The original watercolor paintings are by my daughter-in-law, Glenda Haas. For the preparation of the fruit calendar, I had the help of Mark Cole of Demarest Farms and Glen De Piero of De Piero's Farm. There were numerous contributors for the recipes and acknowledgments are at the end of each recipe. Tajalli Upadhyaya and Irena Yarotsky helped me with the preparation of the manuscript and layout. Dr. Rick Isquith, Glenda Haas, Dr. Hannie Hahn, Dr. Gregory Siragusa, Christopher Rivington, Dr. Pattan Dial, Dr. Doug Eveleigh, and Dr. Scott Mori helped me with proof reading and critique as did my deceased sister Charlotte Schueller. There were many others who helped me with ideas and suggestions.

Copyright © 2013, Royal Fireworks Publishing Co., Inc.
All Rights reserved.

Royal Fireworks Press
First Avenue, PO Box 399
Unionville, NY 10988-0399
(845) 726-4444
Fax: (845) 726-3824
email: mail@rfwp.com
website: rfwp.com

ISBN: 978-0-89824-391-8

Printed and bound in the United States of America using vegetable-based inks on acid-free, recycled paper and environmentally-friendly cover coatings by the Royal Fireworks Printing Co. of Unionville, New York.

Table of Contents

INTRODUCTION 1

Chapter 1: HISTORY OF DOMESTICATION 5

Chapter 2: INDIVIDUAL FRUITS 9

    Apples 9
    Apricots 12
    Avocados 13
    Bananas 14
    Cherries 15
    Citrus Fruits 16
    Dates 20
    Figs 21
    Grapes 22
    Guavas 24
    Kiwi Fruits 25
    Lychees 26
    Mamaey Sapotes 27
    Mangoes 28
    Melons 30
    Nectarines 33
    Papayas 34
    Passion Fruits 35
    Peaches 36
    Pears 38
    Persimmons or Kakis 40
    Pineapples 41
    Plantains 43
    Plums 44
    Pomegranates 46
    Quinces 47
    Star Fruits 48

BERRY FRUITS 49
Blackberries 49
Blueberries 50
Cranberries 52
Currants 53
Gooseberries 54
Raspberries 55
Strawberries 56

Chapter 2: WHAT TO DO WITH THE FRUIT
AFTER YOU GET IT HOME 58

Chapter 3: NUTRITION AND HEALTH 62

Major Constituents 64
Trace Constituents 66

Chapter 4: SOME ASPECTS OF
FRUIT BIOCHEMISTRY AND
THEIR IMPACT ON QUALITY 71

The Ripening Process 71

Recipes from Around the World 74

Appendix 1: METHODS FOR PRESERVING
FRESH FRUIT 99

Appendix 2: FRUIT CALENDAR 102

Appendix 3: SUGGESTIONS FOR ON THE SPOT
EVALUATION 106

About the Author 110

INTRODUCTION

Too often while shopping I see other customers who hardly look at or examine the produce they buy. When I take a moment to check the condition of various fruits, they frequently ask why I do so and what I look for. Fruit is costly; it is disappointing if it does not come up to expectation and worse, has to be discarded, because it is unripe, rotten or off taste.

This book, *Follow Your Nose to the Best Fruit*, is an overview, not all encompassing. I hope that when selecting fruit at the market with more knowledge, it will enhance the enjoyment of this delicious part of our diet. No scientific names or botanical details are given nor is the biochemistry described in detail. It contains what I consider to be the most useful and interesting information for you as a shopper and ultimate consumer. Beyond that, I discuss the health and nutritional aspects of fruits and offer a window to developments in their horticulture and to the past history of consumption. The book emphasizes the fruits with which I have had experience. It is written to help you make your choices at the market and perhaps stimulate your interest in more unusual fruits and varieties.

My interest in fruit is based on several life influences, starting early, for when I was quite young my mother used to take me on her shopping excursions. These were to supply my parents' private hospital with produce for fifty patients and fifty staff members, in addition to providing for our own family needs. The buying occurred at a large marketing center in Munich, Germany. The fruit had been shipped from both Germany and Italy. Because Munich was a trans-shipment point in the days when refrigeration was less efficient, very ripe fruits were separated and sold

Munich at reduced prices as they would not have survived a prolonged further journey.

Other influences were my work experience and educational background. My career as a biological scientist included a need for observation using the senses of vision, smell, taste, and touch. There also was the need to evaluate and compare fruit and other products during my industrial career in the food, beverage, and pharmaceutical industries.

The first and most important factor however, is a love for these wonderful delicacies with which nature so richly has endowed us.

To me, shopping for fruit is both a joy and a challenge. Sometimes, in order to buy the best produce, I may modify my purchasing plans until I can find that fruit which is at its best when I need it. I use my knowledge of maturity of fruits, time of harvest, and the storage periods they have had to endure. The variety is important too as the properties and qualities differ widely. Contrary to advertising claims, size is far less important. If given a choice I may buy smaller fruit, particularly with strawberries and grapes because these are often more flavorful.

I cannot over-emphasize the importance of evaluating fruit by aroma. It can be compared to the way wines are judged by sniffing the bottle and the glass before tasting. People who are particularly good judges of wine should not forget to use this talent when they choose fruit in the market. The same goes for beer experts, as in the brewery aromas are very important when purchasing the raw materials of hops and malt, and also during fermentation and subsequent evaluation of the finished product.

In spite of experience and knowledge there are faults you cannot detect without eating a sample of the produce. This is not always possible before purchase, unless you buy at a farmers' market. Both pears and apples can have internal rot;

melons can be hard and unripe outside and at the same time spoiled inside. Some fruits have 'off' taste originating from the container. Hence, if not too inconvenient, it is better to buy initially a small amount of fruit, and, if it proves to be good, then return for more. Also, if you have to return an unsatisfactory item for credit do not replace it with another fruit from the same batch, but purchase something else for the credit or have the vendor return your money.

The first section of this book is about the individual fruit varieties; the second discusses how to deal with the fruit when you get home; the third considers nutrition and health aspects, the fourth is about some pertinent science for fruit evaluation and ripening, and the fifth gives a short history of the individual fruits and their consumption.

There are three appendices. The first is a calendar showing when specific seasonal fruit is available in northeastern markets. The second appendix illustrates the great variety of fruit used in the culinary sphere with recipes from many different countries. The third is a summary section for immediate use while shopping in a store.

My title, *Follow Your Nose to the Best Fruit*, has a special significance. For no other food selection is the sense of smell as important as for fruit. Upon ripening, agreeable fruit odors are produced by ester formation from fruit acids. Ethyl acetate is a very common component of these esters, and there are other aroma-producing components such as lactones. Off-odors from moldiness or packaging can show you which fruits to shun.

An attractive odor is often the first indicator that the fruit is good and also ripe. The use of the nose is imperative, an essential pre-requisite, for the judgment of peaches, nectarines, apricots, melons, strawberries, and raspberries. For instance, you can stand in front of a bin of melons, and your nose will alert you to the best one ripe enough for early consumption. In addition to the fruits mentioned, your nose will also guide you when evaluating the quality of pears, apples, papayas and mangoes. So following your nose is usually a reliable guide.

Dr. Gerhard J. Haas
Woodcliff Lake, New Jersey

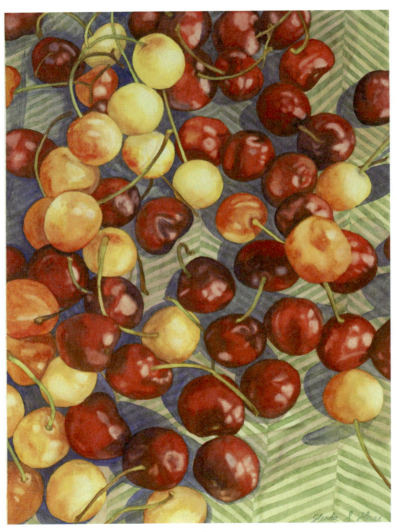

Chapter 1: HISTORY OF DOMESTICATION

When we go to the market and select fruits for the table we usually do not think of the history that has contributed to their availability. There has been a long time period of selection, horticultural progress and consumer preference over the years, all of which have contributed to today's market place.

Fruit derives from trees and other plants domesticated by our ancestors from wild, palatable, and not harmful cultivars. These domesticated fruits made welcome additions to the diet without the need for heat or cooking or much other preparation. Probably the selection of fruit for domestication was also aided by the observation and imitation of the fruit-eating habits of animals such as deer, bear, foxes, bats, monkeys and others. As most of these animals have an acute sense of smell, this certainly helps them choose what is best to eat.

Domestication of fruits goes back for millennia, and interest in their origin is rooted in the legends which are current in many religions and cultures: the apple in the Garden of Eden, the apple in the story of Snow White and the story of Wilhelm Tell. Apples and pineapples are a symbol of fertility in Greek, Roman and other cultures. In China the apple is a symbol of peace. There are many legends and stories about golden apples whose consumption leads to eternal life and immortality.

The sayings 'the apple of his eye' and 'an apple a day keeps the doctor away' both speak to the special desirable qualities of the apple. The pear, the pomegranate and the fig also feature in mythology.

It is remarkable, however, how little is known about domestication of even the most popular fruits. The following table shows some of the locations and dates for certain fruits. For apples, pears, and bananas there is good documentation of the wild species from which they were developed into their presently available larger and sweeter versions. In several other cases they were further improved in a second or even third country, so in these instances a clear-cut location and time of domestication is not possible.

Fruit	Where Domesticated	Date
Apples	Multicentric (Central Asia, Europe)	800 BC (Greece)
Apricots	Central and South East Asia	2000 BC
Avocados	Central America	5000 BC
Bananas	Malaysia, Guinea, Southeast Asia, and India	600 BC - 300 BC
Blackberries	U.S.	Contemporary
Blueberries	U.S.	Contemporary
Cherries	Egypt, China, Italy, Greece	100 BC - Rome
Dates	Middle East	3000 BC
Figs	Near East	9000 BC
Grapes	Southwest Asia	4000 BC
Grapefruits	West Indies, South East Asia	18th Century AD
Kiwis	China	1900 AD
Lemons	India	800 BC

Mangoes	India, Malaysia	4000 BC
Oranges	China, India	2000 BC
Papayas	Central America	
Peaches	Central Asia, China	2000 BC
Pears	Northern France, Rome, China	
Pineapples	Brazil/Paraguay	Probably before 1300 AD
Plums	Iraq and later improved by the Romans	
Pomegranates	Iran	3500 BC
Watermelons	Near East	4000 BC

Plant domestication, Table of Dates and Places by K. Kris Hirst

With the improvements in propagation methodology there was a big upswing in domestication. Seeds of many fruit varieties do not breed "true". Often seeds from a larger or sweeter cultivar may not yield progeny with those desirable properties. The following methods came into general use: cuttings, layering and particularly use of grafting where plants with desirable properties can be grafted onto rootstock of wild (not domesticated) plants. This greatly advanced the possibilities of fruit breeding. These methods were developed several millennia ago and led to our large number of palatable fruit varieties.

In recent times our knowledge of genetics has enabled plant breeders to develop new varieties such as crosses between different fruits like apricots and plums. The *pluot* is a hybrid between apricots and plums developed in several steps by crosses and back-crosses. It is round and resembles a plum, very juicy, dark purple, sweet and flavorful. The color of the flesh varies between different varieties, many of which have made the stores. *Aprium* and *plumcote* are other plum-apricot hybrids which are at times commercially available. Other crosses between types of berries and involving apples are occasionally available.

Fruit hybrids also can occur in nature. Some of the fruits that are familiar to us originate from hybrids developed centuries ago. For instance, grapefruit is such a hybrid of orange and pomelo.

Recently produced hybrids are usually more expensive than the individual varieties, thus profitable for the seller and a premium is charged to the consumer for the added technology. The world of fruit use is dynamic. Preferences come and go and are aided by changes in technology and molded by lifestyle, fads, and medical pronouncements.

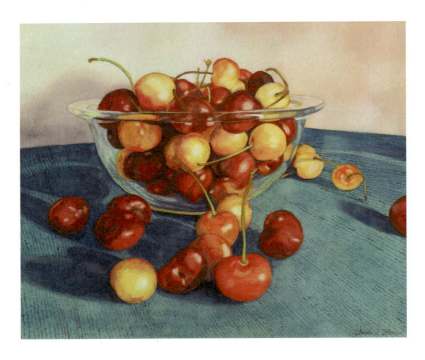

Chapter 2: INDIVIDUAL FRUITS

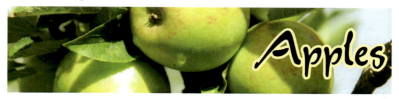

The apple is one of the most popular fruits. They should be firm, without bruises or other physical damage; pips should be black; in most varieties there is a good aroma that becomes more noticeable upon cutting. The best fruit is available during the harvest season for that particular variety; the vitamin levels are at their peak when the fruit is the freshest because these levels decay with time. With prolonged storage many apple varieties become softer and lose aroma and flavor. When this reduction of quality becomes evident, I substitute with other fruits until apples imported from south of the Equator become available. In March you can purchase imported apples and pears that are mostly of good quality.

Depending on the season, there are numerous varieties of apple available and they all differ in flavor, aroma, size and texture. Tables 1 and 2 should be useful in helping you choose what to buy; not all apples available in any one locality are mentioned and new varieties appear in the stores almost every year. In Table 1, separation of apples into classifications based on texture is partially subjective and so is the classification for utility in Table 2.

Popular and available apple varieties vary with region and country. For example, in England and New Zealand "Cox's Orange Pippin" is a favorite, while in Germany "Lederapfel" and "Reinette" are popular varieties. If an apple is dropped in handling, it should be eaten right away as it almost invariably bruises in a short time.

New apple varieties are developed and breeders constantly try to improve some of the less favored apple varieties; for instance, Cortland apples have become firmer, appealing to more customers while previously they were almost too soft.

So many people only purchase one or two varieties of apples without enjoying the many different flavors, aromas, and textures that are available. The most frequently used apples by far in hotels for example, are Golden and Red Delicious varieties because of their excellent keeping qualities, but this can become monotonous to their guests.

TABLE 1: *Some of the Apple Varieties Arranged According to Apparent Hardness. Of course, hardness is also influenced by ripeness: an apple picked early is usually harder than the one harvested later; stored apples gradually become softer even when storage takes place in the refrigerator, only more slowly.*

HARD	MEDIUM	SOFT
Fuji	Braeburn	Cortland
Granny Smith	Gala	Ida Red
Jazz	Ginger Golden	Rome
Mutsu	Golden Delicious	
Winesap	Jonathan	
Honey Crisp	Lady Apples	
	McIntosh	
	Macoun	
	Paula Red	
	Red Delicious	

TABLE 2: Optimum Apple Varieties for the Following Food Applications:

FRESH EATING	APPLE SAUCE	BAKING	FREEZING
Cortland	Empire	Iowa Gold	Ida Red
Ginger Golden	Golden Delicious	Golden Delicious	Golden Delicious
Golden Delicious	Ida Red	Granny Smith	Mutsu
Empire	Jonathan	Northern Spy	Northern Spy
Jonagold	Mutsu	Rome	
Macoun	Macintosh		
Mutsu	Northern Spy		
Northern Spy			
Winesap			

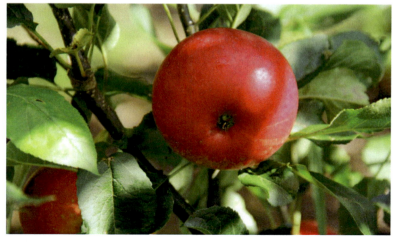

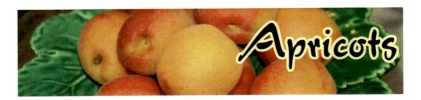

Apricots

Aroma is the most important indicator of flavor and ripeness of apricots. A golden color is often also a sign of good quality. The apricot is particularly sweet and excellent for eating fresh as well as cooked in numerous recipes.

Early and late crops are best in my experience as they have the good aroma that is essential for palatability; larger fruit are often inferior to smaller ones. Do not buy when too hard or unripe or when too mushy, as apricots ripen very unevenly. Be careful to check the fruit for spoilage starting as brown spots which can happen very rapidly. Do not buy if there are off smells from packaging material such as cardboard.

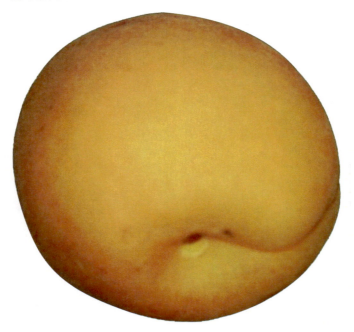

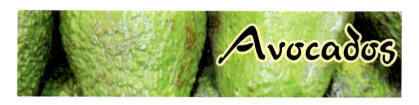

Avocados

My favorite of the two most popular varieties is the Hass Avocado because of its nutty delicate flavor (and not because it is similar to my name). Florida avocados are larger, but in my opinion, the flavor is somewhat inferior. Avocados should not be over-ripe and too soft when purchased. Sometimes there are dark colored islands in the skin, which can mar appearance and flavor. Avocados ripen well on the household counter, but they can lose quality when stored too long in the refrigerator. Also they are very sensitive to bruises when dropped or knocked, turning black at the injured area.

When cutting an avocado, exposure to air should be minimized as it will go black. If you are not going to use all of it at once, cut the part to be eaten inside an open zip-lock bag and then close the bag to keep the unused portion from excessive air exposure.

Avocados are high in mono-unsaturated fat, which is healthy and can replace other less healthful fats such as butter and margarine when preparing many types of sandwiches.

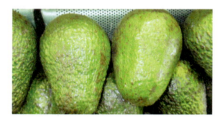

Best storage depends on the ripeness when buying and the time interval for consumption. If the avocado is on the soft side, refrigerate till time of use, otherwise let it ripen on the counter to the desired texture.

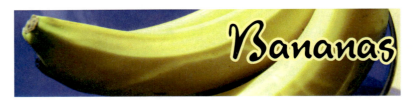

Bananas

Bananas ripen well in the home and hence should not be bought overripe. The stem end should preferably be slightly green at the time of purchase and there should be no black spots. If the banana has freckle-like spots, it is overripe and should not be bought. Some bananas may have soft spots and you should avoid these.

Bananas produce ethylene, one of the ripening hormones; so each banana as it gets ripe accelerates the ripening of other nearby bananas. Another sign of over-ripeness is a strong banana odor. Ripening can be speeded by storage in a paper bag. The organically grown bananas which I have tried did appear to have a taste advantage over regular bananas.

There are many varieties in different countries. When I lived in Cuba there were more than ten, but here in the U.S., there are usually just three or four types available. One is a very small banana; the other has red skin. Both show some taste differences and have their fans. Red bananas originate from Costa Rica, which exported them to other South-American countries. Several varieties are available throughout most of South America and sometimes available in U.S. specialty fruit stores.

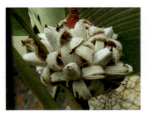

Bananas are a sweet fruit with appreciable starch content which is greater in the less ripe bananas. This content decreases as some of it is converted into sugar. Bananas are very easily peeled and the skin is an excellent container, making them extremely popular and good to take in lunch boxes, picnics and hikes.

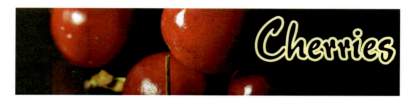

Cherries

Wild cherry trees, from which sweet cherries were cultivated, are widespread in Europe and Asia. Cherry pits have been found in Bronze Age settlements and the first mention of cherry cultivation was in Rome during the first century BC.

The blossoms of cherry trees are one of the most beautiful harbingers of spring and the whole family of cherry trees has many members with such exquisite blooms. However, many of these trees have small, bitter fruits with little flesh, but are well liked by birds.

High in antioxidants, cherries are some of the most consistently good fruits. There are several varieties on the market: Bing cherries which have to be firm to keep well; Rainier Cherries which are pale, sweeter, more perishable and usually more expensive. Some of the local cherry varieties are very flavorful and less costly than the Bing, unless you are living on the West Coast where they are grown. Sour cherries are mostly local, excellent for compote and for baking and in desserts, but are quite perishable, and should be used as soon as you can. They are true to their name "sour"; thus eating them depends on personal preference.

Cherries must not be stored for too long and if there is more than one spoiled (moldy or decayed) cherry in a count of twenty, or a noticeably soft one, do not buy; the others in the package will turn soft rapidly and will become inedible and rotten. Often this softening precedes the decay and turns the cherries from a treat to a decayed fruit. Cherries should not have wrinkled skin! It is best to store all cherries in the refrigerator to preserve them longer.

Citrus Fruits

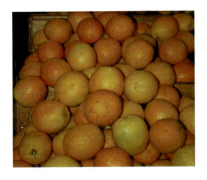

Fruits of the citrus family are well known: oranges, lemons and grapefruit are used in most households, while tangerines, clementines, mandarins, temple oranges, limes, pomelos, kumquats, mineolas and other citrus fruits are frequently offered in our markets. They all have a juicy, refreshing taste, and contain pectin, sugars, Vitamin C and citric acid.

Some markets sell freshly squeezed orange juice and so do many restaurants. Industrially produced orange juice, which is sold in bottles or in cartons, is a very large article of commerce and orange juice futures are traded on the commodity exchange. There are several different processes to produce this juice, some based on first preparing a concentrate. In years when juice is in short supply because of climatic conditions, Brazil has frequently acted as a good second supplier for orange juice. However, in such years, the price of juice usually increases.

It is very important that all citrus fruit is fresh when you buy it—and how to achieve this depends to a large extent on where you live. In those states and/or countries where oranges grow, you can buy them freshly picked, whilst elsewhere you are dependent on the shipper and wholesaler. Wholesalers often store the fruit for long periods, sometimes treating them with antifungals or coloring agents.

U.S.A.-grown fruits are the freshest during the following periods; grapefruits: December to April, lemons: November to March, oranges: November to February, and tangerines: November through December.

When using citrus rind in recipes it should be exclusively from organic sources as most of the non-organically grown citrus fruits contain wax, color, and/or fungicides. Even when you taste citrus samples at markets you should keep this in mind.

The best fruits are bought as close to harvest time as possible, especially as the Vitamin C content decreases steadily after picking, even when refrigerated. Good oranges and grapefruit have a tight skin and are heavy for their size; reject any with loose skin or soft areas. Color of the skin is not important; brown, green, or almost black areas are not signs of poor quality; in many cases, to enhance sales appeal, the skin of oranges is artificially colored by the grower. Look out for dark black spots at the navel area of California oranges as these may be an indication of fungal infection and decay.

Many of the criteria above are also valid for other citrus fruits. In temple oranges, clementines, and some other fruits the skin may be looser without any concurrent faults. Blood oranges are rather sweet but otherwise do not, in my opinion, deserve the special premium that is demanded for them.

Citrus fruits must never freeze, whether this happens in the field or in the freezer.

When making orange juice, be aware that one bad orange even in a large quantity of juice affects the whole batch and may make it undrinkable.

It is difficult to evaluate the quality of citrus fruit while in the store. Once you have tried one, the quality of oranges should be judged by juiciness and flavor; the *albedo* (the 'white under the outer skin') should not be thick and should be easily removable from the flesh. The skin surrounding the individual sections must not be too fibrous. They should be sweet and not dried out.

The aroma of an unpeeled orange in the market place is often faint and at times even nonexistent and not necessarily a good guide for purchase in this case.

Fruits with thin skin are juicier. If they are pointed at the stem end it is a sign that they may be thick skinned with less juice.

Today most oranges have very few or no seeds. This was accomplished by the breeding of seedless varieties. The same has been achieved with grapefruits, but there are still more grapefruits with seeds than oranges.

The most plentiful supply of eating oranges is from California, with Valencia and Navel varieties. Florida is the main supplier of juice oranges but it also has some good Navel oranges. Brazil, Chile, Israel, South Africa, Morocco, Australia, Spain and Italy are important competitors in the world markets and some oranges from these countries are also imported to the U.S. In addition to Florida and California, Texas is an important supplier of grapefruit; most of the other citrus fruits come from California and Florida and the U.S. competitors mentioned above.

The lemon is a rather acidic citrus fruit widely grown, particularly in warm regions of the United States and Italy.

It became well-known when lemons were found to prevent scurvy in sailors who had no other fresh fruit in their diet.

When purchasing lemons they should have tight skin and be heavy for their size. For maximum juice yield the fruit should be at room temperature when squeezed. Also the lemon can be rolled with a little pressure or it can be briefly microwaved for good yield of juice. Lemons are rarely consumed fresh, but lemon juice is added to many hot and cold drinks, meats, fish and desserts, and also added to fruit salads and some other salads where its acidity will prevent darkening of many fruits as well as of mushrooms.

Limes are small, sour fruits with green skin and lots of juice; it is used in some beverages and recipes instead of lemon.

Limes and lemons have an aroma discernible in the store and this is an indicator of freshness and taste.

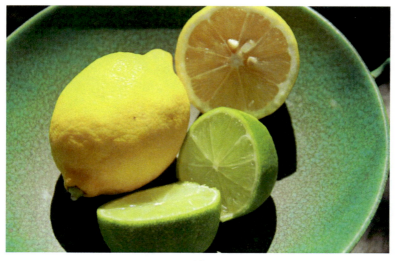

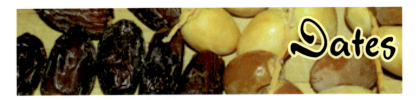

Dates

Dates, the fruits of the date palm, are one of the oldest domesticated fruits. They are cultivated in arid areas such as the Middle East where the palms have to be irrigated. By far the biggest exporters are the Arab countries, North Africa and Turkey, but dates are also grown in the U.S. in California and some other western states. In my experience they appear to be somewhat more popular in Europe than in the United States, and in Germany and England they are often included in seasonal gift packages.

Dates appear to the palate very much like a candied fruit, because they are low in water content, very sweet and high in carbohydrates, with about 25 calories per date. Besides their high sugar content, dates have nutritionally valuable constituents, particularly fiber, Vitamin C, and potassium.

There are dry dates, semi-moist dates, and fresh dates ranging from brown to black depending on the variety. Fresh dates are seasonal, crunchy, juicy, but less sweet than the dried.

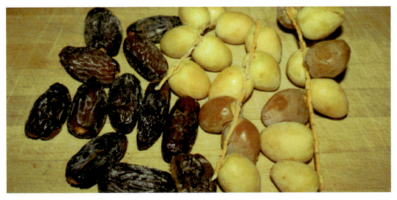

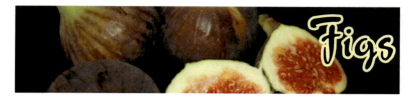

Figs

Figs are popular in the dried state all year, and in late summer and early fall fresh figs are available almost everywhere, usually in two varieties, green and black. Critics have different taste preferences but all agree that there are excellent varieties of each color, and I personally do not detect a characteristically distinct flavor difference for either variety. All are high in sugar and have appreciable caloric content.

The color of the flesh varies; it can be deep purple to golden brown. Fresh figs are very sensitive and have a soft skin which is easily injured; before buying check for injuries and bruises. Figs are superior when you can pick them from a tree and eat them then and there. In some climatic areas it is hard to get them to ripen before the frost comes in the fall.

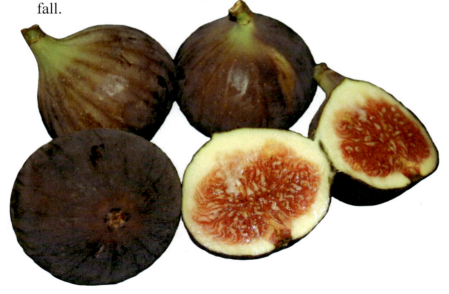

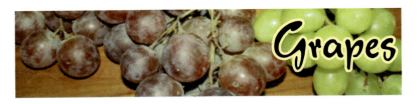

Grapes

Different consumers like grapes of different color: green, red or black. I enjoy green grapes most for their flavor and sometimes for a pleasant crunchiness. Size is not important for flavor. Seeded grapes are not liked by many people.

A sample grape should always be evaluated for flavor and texture (guard for toughness of the skin), also it should be checked to see if it is beginning to spoil at the stem end.

The flavor of grapes is made up of sweetness, some tartness, and the effect of appealing volatiles such as esters. Usually it is best not to buy grapes if too many have been dislodged from the stem. Concord grapes, available in the late summer to fall, are grown predominantly locally and have a much stronger taste than other grape varieties; they are usually purple and have pits. These grapes are also available in Europe, particularly in northern Italy. Their taste is both sweet and tart.

Caution: In some people, the gum is sensitive to grapes and they may lead to canker sores when large amounts are eaten.

Grapes are the fruit most used in wine fermentation. Wine grapes are selected for the taste they give to specific wines and good wine grapes are not necessarily best for eating fresh. Non-alcoholic juice from both red and green grapes is popular in Europe. There are many different types of grapes both in size and flavor as well as in the presence or absence of seeds and in the thickness of the skin. Also the red grapes contain a chemical compound called reservatol which is claimed to be beneficial for the heart.

When grapes are dried to produce raisins there are also wide differences in the quality and type of the raisins produced.

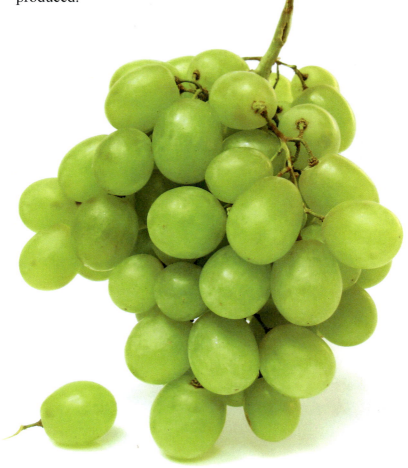

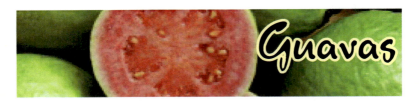

Guavas

The Guava, grown throughout the Caribbean, in Northern and Western India and in Indonesia, is eaten as fresh fruit and in desserts, juice and jam.

There is a dessert in Cuba, which I found very appealing, "casco de guava." It appeared to me to have a taste like candied fruit. In India, guavas are mostly eaten with their skin and sliced. The slices are sprinkled with salt and red chili powder.

Guava is at times available in the markets and the species 'apple guava' is the most popular type. It is usually green to yellow but a red cultivar also exists. Other species of guava are cultivated in some countries.

Guava is very high in pectin and rich in potassium and Vitamin C; the red varieties are also rich in antioxidants. Guava leaves are being studied for medical applications particularly for diabetes and cancer.

The fruit is eaten whole or peeled. Even though the guava is hard, it has a sweet taste.

Ripeness is judged by a good aroma, a yellowish green and soft skin; an unripe fruit is often purely green in color.

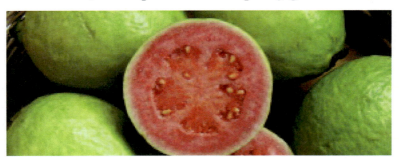

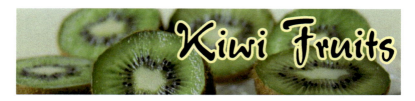

Kiwi Fruits

The Kiwi fruit is a comparatively recent addition to today's available fruits and is named after the Kiwi bird, the national bird of New Zealand, where 20th century commercial production began. Originally a native to China, it only became familiar and popular in the U.S. after the Second World War when improvements in transportation made imports possible. Before that it had been referred to as the Chinese gooseberry because the taste reminded some people of the taste of gooseberry; however the two fruits are not related.

It is a brown hairy fruit with green and yellow flesh and a refreshing, slightly astringent, taste. It will keep several weeks at room temperature and several months in the refrigerator.

Its color and appearance make it useful in fruit salads but it will liquefy gelatin and certain milk-based products.

Kiwis should be soft but not mushy before eating. Kiwis have particularly good nutritional properties and are known for their high Vitamin C content. Kiwi fruit is reasonably priced and available in markets for most of the year. Italy has overtaken New Zealand as the largest Kiwi producer and cultivation has also increased in the U.S. and several other countries.

Caution: It contains a proteolytic enzyme and can cause canker sores in people who are sensitive.

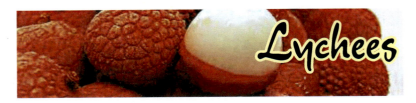

Lychees

Lychees can be traced in Chinese records to at least 2000 B.C. They are predominantly cultivated in the tropical and sub-tropical regions of China and South East Asia, where they also grow wild. They have also been cultivated in India and the United States.

They are usually eaten as a fresh fruit because when preserved much of the aroma of the fruit is lost. However, canned products: lychee juice, lychee jam and dried lychees, are commercially available everywhere all the year round.

Lychee fruit grows on 10-20 feet high trees with a copious yield. From a distance the fruit on the tree resembles large raspberries. They have a red inedible skin concealing a flavourful, fleshy interior. Numerous different cultivars are being grown and these differ considerably in appearance and flavor. Lychees are a component of many Chinese recipes. Lychee juice is a popular drink and is also used in cocktails. Lychees keep well when stored in the refrigerator.

When buying fresh lychees in the store, the fruit should be pink and not green and have a slight give when pressed with a finger, but they must not be too soft indicating over ripeness.

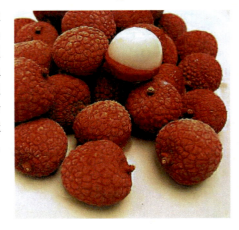

Mamaey Sapotes

Mamaey sapote is very popular in Cuba and the other Caribbean islands, and also in India where it's called Chikoo. It can be purple or brown, grows on trees, and has a strong, unusual, sweet taste.

The fruit should be eaten only when completely ripe, which you can test by aroma and softness.

It can be eaten in the fresh state after peeling and also used in milk shakes, or as a component of desserts such as ice cream. Fresh and canned fruits are obtainable in Mexican and Indian grocery stores and, at times, in certain fruit markets.

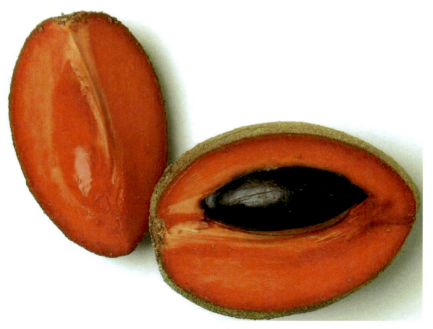

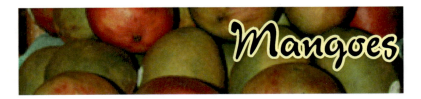

Mangoes

Mangoes are one of the most popular fruits in the world and they are consumed very frequently in the Caribbean countries, Florida, and also in India. Many people in the U.S. are not familiar with mangoes but they miss so much if they don't try them. They were grown originally in only tropical countries, but their range has very much expanded and there are many sub-varieties.

When purchasing a mango the texture is important. The fruit should not be totally hard but also not too soft.

It is difficult to judge at what point of hardness the mango should be eaten. While it should be soft, excessive softness goes hand in hand with internal rot. A mango with any internal spoilage is usually inedible even after you remove the spoiled part as the whole fruit then has an off-taste. The aroma of the mango is sometimes an indicator

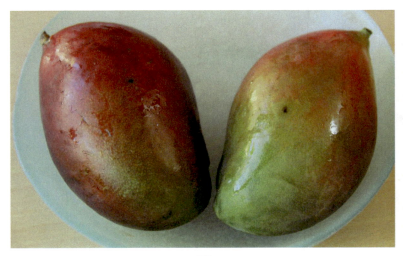

of quality. They are at times stringy and fibrous, but this is not predictable without cutting them open. The skin color is almost immaterial. I have eaten completely green mangoes. If they are soft to the touch they can have good aroma and taste.

Eating mangoes can be quite tricky. They have a large pit and are very slippery when peeled. The first mango I peeled when I was on shipboard, slipped overboard out of my hands when I tried to eat it. Now I have learned better as it is best to cut it into sections off the pit and peel the sections individually.

I understand that in India there are now different kinds of mangoes commercially available, particularly the Kesar variety, but I am only familiar with what is available in Cuba, the U.S., and Central Europe. In the U.S., in addition to the usual Caribbean type, you can also at times buy the so-called Champagne mangoes which are less rounded in shape and in my opinion have a better taste.

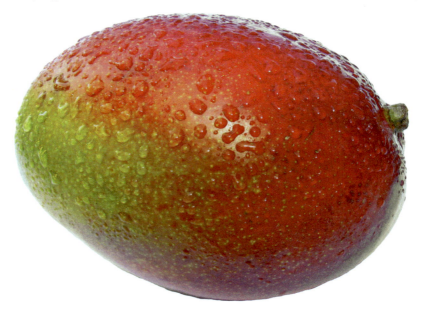

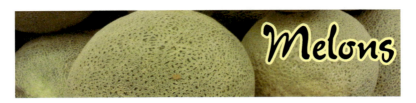

Melons

Melons can vary tremendously in quality from superb to having a strong metallic or perfume like off-taste. In stores you may find the following melon varieties, in approximate order of availability: Cantaloupe, Honeydew, Watermelon, Crenshaw, Casaba, Galia and Persian.

The cantaloupe melon is difficult to evaluate as to eating quality. It is available all year and when out of season (probably obtained out of storage or from different countries) it often has little taste. In season it is aromatic and delightful. When you buy, consider for which future meal you are buying the melon; it is hard to predict when it will be at its optimum ripeness.

Usually, when slightly soft to the touch at the smooth (stem) side cantaloupe melons will ripen at room temperature within 24-48 hours. This is when the aroma develops.

When at the time of purchase they feel hard it may take two to five days, but occasionally the melon may not even ripen in two weeks or more showing that it was picked too soon.

Early good aroma is an advance indicator of an appealing taste experience and it is indeed risky to select melons without any good aroma at all. A slightly golden color of the skin is also a good desirable.

Many cantaloupes do not develop the sweet and aromatic odor and some can even have off odors or chemical odors particularly when purchased out of season. Sometimes cantaloupes grown away from the western states can be satisfactory, but their flavor is usually not as good.

Honeydew melons can be more flavorful than all the other melons when ripe and of good aroma, but most are hard when arriving at the market and it is unpredictable when they will ripen.

I have had to keep this fruit for five or six weeks till edible and at times it never ripens. If you have guests on a certain day delay in ripening can be very annoying. "Golden flesh melons", a hybrid of the honeydew, often have a particularly good aroma and flavor.

To summarize, it is somewhat difficult to have a good honeydew melon available when you need it—but when you do have one, it is a delight. With both melons the motto of "following your nose" is invaluable and enables you to pick out the best melon in a whole batch. Neither cantaloupe nor honeydew is enjoyable when eaten too hard and without flavor.

For both cantaloupe and honeydew, one has to check for deep bruises, which could indicate internal rot. Crenshaw melons when available are fairly reliably good and of good aroma and texture indicating ripeness and a good eating experience. When hard they usually ripen in a few days. Casaba and Galia melons should also be eaten when ripe.

With Galia melons, which are generally more expensive, the aroma is not always reliable and I have had some specimens which seem to have good aroma and yet very little flavor.

Large, juicy watermelons are popular at picnics. They are often sweet but frequently low in flavor. Though seedless watermelons can be purchased, in most watermelons the seeds are plentiful and in ripe fruit are loose and dispersed. The seeds are supposed to have beneficial effects on the prostate and urinary system and are often eaten for that purpose.

The flesh of watermelons is usually pink to crimson red, but there are also varieties with yellow flesh.

Ripeness can be estimated by the sound when knocking against the melon with the knuckle; a higher pitch indicates ripeness.

Another method is to look at the rings around the skin of the watermelon. When ripe the rings are interrupted, where the melon lies on the ground and the color in that area of the melon is yellow to yellow-brown.

Before purchase, the melon should be visually inspected, as it should be hard and without soft spots; also it should be dry at the stem end.

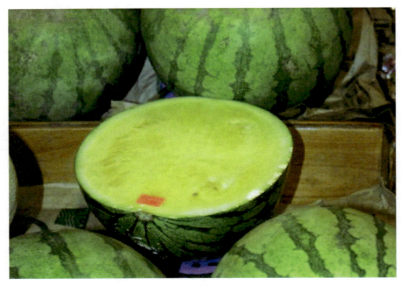

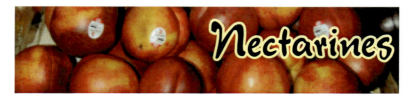

Nectarines

Nectarines should be bought when ripe, meaning that they are slightly tender to the touch, but not discolored or with broken skin; they also should be aromatic.

In my opinion, the aroma is the number one indicator for the choice of this excellent fruit.

The best nectarines are bought at the peak of the season, which is from the middle of July till the end of August; if they are picked too early, aroma and ripeness may never develop.

So-called "tree ripe" fruits are often picked too early and not ripe at all. Towards the end of the season the skin may be leathery and the flesh mealy. One should never purchase nectarines with leathery skin.

Both white and yellow nectarines can be excellent and locally grown nectarines often are particularly desirable. Chilean nectarines, available in our markets in January, are often of good quality but do not ripen uniformly and deteriorate as the season progresses to become quite tasteless. When you buy these nectarines, ripe conditions and good aroma are particularly important to assure a satisfying experience.

However, some unripe fruits will ripen to good quality when bought and then stored at home at room temperature. I have not found a sure way to predict which unripe fruit will become good and which will not spoil before it can ripen fully, so purchasing ripe fruit is the best if you want to be sure.

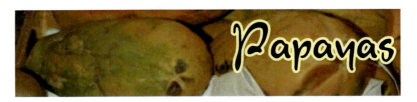

Papayas

The popularity of papayas has increased greatly in recent years. The imports from Hawaii and from the Caribbean are quite different from one another. The Caribbean Papaya is yellow brown and usually weighs several pounds. The Hawaiian Papaya is green to green yellow and weighs one to two pounds.

As they bruise easily when ripe, papayas are shipped unripe. They ripen and become soft when stored at room temperature in the store or at home.

When purchasing papayas avoid bruised fruit; Caribbean papayas at times have mold on the skin, which is undesirable. Papayas usually have many round black seeds, but recently some seedless varieties have been developed. The seeds are reported to be edible but no one I know eats them, and I lived two years in Cuba, where papaya is eaten very frequently. The papaya has a proteolytic enzyme, papain, and can be used in marinades. This enzyme is also used to prevent protein hazes in beer. Fresh papaya is consumed cold like melon and is often used in fruit salads and desserts as well as in savory dishes. The fruit is rich in Vitamin C, A and potassium.

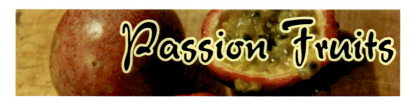

Passion Fruits

Passion fruit is from a tropical plant cultivated commercially in India, New Zealand, Central and South American countries as well as in California, Florida, Hawaii, Australia and Israel. It was named by catholic missionaries who gave it some religious connection. There are two varieties of passion fruit, the most frequently eaten is purple and has juicy flesh and many seeds. Passion fruit, when ripe, falls to the ground; the skin is still hard and the color deep purple; at this stage, the passion fruit can be eaten.

The fruit is cut open longitudinally and the flesh, which is the edible portion, is scooped out and eaten fresh or used in recipes.

The sweetness is enhanced if the fruit is stored at room temperature until it wrinkles. Then, at this stage, it is best moved to the refrigerator till the time of consumption.

It can also be frozen for later use. The juice is very popular in many countries and is best when collected at this wrinkled and high sugar level stage. A much larger species of passion fruit exists which is yellow and mainly used for juice. Passion fruit and passion fruit juice are often added to desserts. Passion fruit has health applications such as for lowering blood pressure and as a source of Vitamin C.

The passion fruit plant has pretty flowers and the plants are at times available, particularly in England, for indoor decorative purposes.

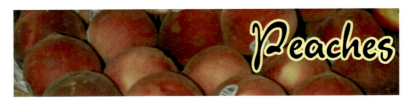

Peaches

Similar considerations as for nectarines hold for peaches. Aroma is the most important. Best if fruit is bought when there is a slight give to the flesh when you press with your finger; at that time the aroma should have developed and imminent ripening is indicated.

Some peaches, especially early in the season, have a deep groove or indentation going down the side of the peach. This may indicate that the peach has a broken pit, which can be deleterious to the flavor, due to very bitter components, including traces of cyanide.

Also such peaches may have small pit fragments in the flesh. This signals that you might better postpone your purchase until fruit without such indentation is available, or otherwise proceed with caution.

While there are many varieties of peaches, the main categories are Clingstone and Freestone varieties. The flesh of the Clingstone, as the name implies, stubbornly clings to the pit. Freestone peaches are more popular as the flesh can be easily removed from the pit. Clingstone peaches ripen earlier than Freestone varieties, usually in mid to late May. Freestones ripen in mid June through late July.

When the peach is truly ripe, the skin is more easily peeled off the flesh. I thoroughly recommend peeling, as pesticides are difficult to remove from the fuzzy surface of the peach by washing. When the fruit is easy to peel, it is a sign that prime peach time is here, which gives the best opportunity to make peach pies, jam or compote. Excellent fruit should be available through September.

Late in the season peaches can become mealy and tasteless just as happens with nectarines, probably from being stored too long. (This usually occurs after September 20 in New Jersey and New York and then it is best to wait for Chilean imports or otherwise for next year's crop.)

White flesh peaches are often particularly flavorful. During the last few years a new peach variety "donut peaches" has been developed. They are very sweet but also carry a premium price.

Before leaving this discussion on peaches, I want to warn you that it is particularly important that the fruit is ripe and ready to eat at the time of purchase.

Recently, I did not examine a basket of Georgia peaches well enough. The top three peaches were excellent; while the bottom ones were not ripe; these never ripened when held at room temperature for five days at which time they became moldy. Obviously, they had been picked too early. This happened on June 20th well into the season of peach availability in stores. Equal caution in selection of fruit is necessary when picking nectarines or apricots.

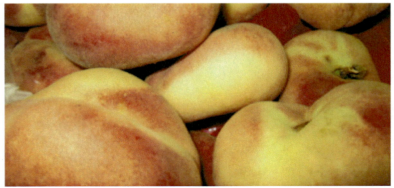

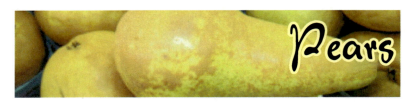

Pears

Different varieties of pears are different not only in appearance but also in properties. The following pears are available in markets for much of the year: Bartlett, Anjou, Comice, Bosc, Forelli, Seckel, Red, Thomson (available for a short period)

Each variety has a distinct appearance, flavor, texture, keeping quality, and size. All pears go through a process called climacteric. This process will be discussed later in the book, when the difference between climacteric and non-climacteric fruits will be explained.

At room temperature pears remain very firm for a time and then ripen and become soft rapidly. In some varieties this process progresses so rapidly that the change from good eating to over-ripeness, softness and rotting can all occur within one or two days.

Hence at the first appreciable softness the pears should be moved from room temperature to the refrigerator so as to slow this process, but certain varieties continue to deteriorate even after they have been moved into the refrigerator. It is also usually best to buy pears slightly unripe and then let them ripen in the home, checking them every day for the right time to place in the refrigerator. Anjou pears are the most resistant to rotting, while

Comice are very sensitive. Seckel pears have to be eaten when they are just ripe and give very slightly when pressed with the finger; then they can be excellent; they are not at their best any more when the pears are really soft. Small eastern Seckel pears are often better tasting than the larger western variety. Bosc pears should be bought early in their season. Later in the season they are at times black and rotten inside, even before they are soft enough to eat and show visible decay on the outside. In addition to this rotting they can also turn mealy.

Taylor pears are a more recent addition to pear varieties, and are at times available as imports from New Zealand. They are very juicy and tasty with a russet skin; usually they are a little more expensive than other varieties. Peckam pears are very similar to Bartlett pears. In Europe several other pear varieties are available but are not exported to the U.S.

Some pear varieties at times get gritty or grainy which can lead to an unpleasant sensation. This happens particularly frequently with the following varieties: Red, Bosc, Anjou, and Seckel, arranged in order of frequency of this phenomenon. I personally like Comice pears the best because they are very juicy and usually have no graininess.

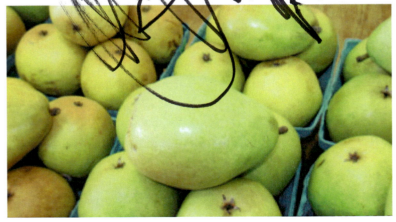

Persimmons or Kakis

When I was a child in Germany, my parents occasionally had an orange colored fruit in their fruit bowl. It was a persimmon and supposed to be a special treat, but I found it insipid and cloyingly sweet. After many years I met the fruit again in our U.S. markets. They vary widely in taste and astringency.

The degree of ripeness is most important. Unripe fruit is so astringent that it is inedible. Ripening reduces the tannins, which cause the astringency, but in some varieties it still remains very apparent.

The history of the persimmon goes back over many centuries and it is known that they were eaten in ancient Greece and by Native Americans. Large crops are grown in the Orient and Brazil, but some persimmons are also grown in the United States. In Mitchell, Indiana, there is even a persimmon festival.

Persimmons are best eaten fresh, particularly the variety Fuyu. But they are also used dried and cooked, often as an ingredient in pies and puddings. Sharon fruit, developed in the Sharon valley of Israel, is an improved variety of persimmon and is seedless.

Caution! Consuming too many unripe persimmons can lead to dangerous digestive problems. Persimmons should always be eaten after the removal of the skin, because eating unpeeled fruit has also been reported to cause digestive difficulties.

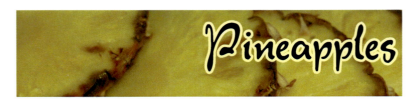

Pineapples

The popularity of pineapple is due to its pleasant sweet acidic taste and its availability all year around. For eating, the pineapple must be at the right stage of ripeness but not overripe or rotten.

One criterion for selecting a pineapple is how easily the leaves are removed when pulling them from the pineapple. If this cannot be done easily the pineapple is not ripe enough; when it can be done the pineapple is probably ready.

Another quality criterion is the odor at the bottom end of the pineapple. It should smell slightly like a good pineapple; it will develop a bad odor when it is starting to rot, usually at the bottom end. A pineapple which is ready will also yield when the lower part of the fruit is tested for "give" with the finger.

The larger the pineapple the greater is the proportion of edible fruit. Pineapples are native to South America but are mainly imported from Hawaii, and the Caribbean. Candied dried pineapple is often sold and popular with hikers; pineapple juice is on the menus of many restaurants, and pineapple is often served with meat.

Caution! Some people's gums and tongue are sensitive to the proteolytic enzyme called bromelin in pineapples and they can get canker sores from eating pineapple too frequently.

The pineapple was domesticated at the Brazil-Paraguay border and spread throughout South and Central America. It was brought to Europe by Christopher Columbus and from there it spread throughout the world.

The name pineapple comes from its resemblance to a pine cone, but in some countries such as Germany, and in France, the name is *ananas* after the botanical name *Ananas comosus*. It is particularly popular in the Philippines where several legends have developed around it and it is grown commercially on a large scale there and in Hawaii. These, as well as the Caribbean countries, are the main exporters to the U.S.; Costa Rica, particularly, has a large export business. Many of the pineapples sold in the U.S. are low acid hybrids, which were developed in Hawaii.

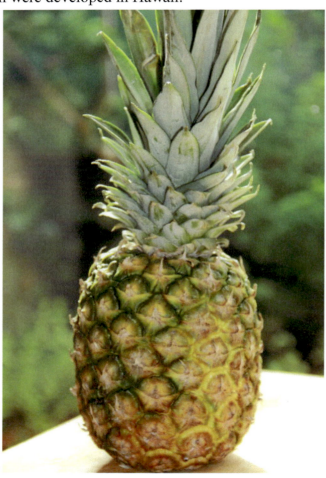

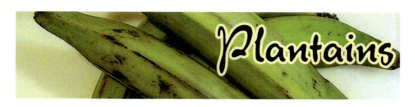

Plantains

The plantain, a native of India, is used mainly for cooking, often fried or baked. While related and with a similar shape to the banana, it is high in starch and low in sugar. It is especially popular in Caribbean countries where it is eaten as a substitute for potato. Unripe plantains are also used to make chips or porridge.

With ripening, the skin color changes from green to yellow and black, but the interior color remains creamy yellow to light pink.

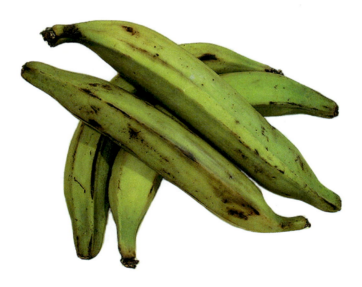

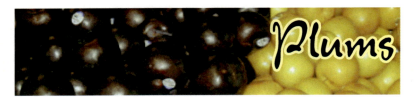

Plums

There are many varieties of plum and every year there seems to be new ones. Most are blue or purple, but others are red, green, or yellow.

When buying plums, it is best if you can buy just one or two first and taste them, because some varieties are very sour and others quite sweet.

Many are hard and do not ripen well, rotting on one side while remaining unripe on the other. I only buy those plums that are ready to eat immediately.

I particularly shy away from blue, red or black round plums when they are hard, as often they do not ripen properly. When these plums have small white spots giving a mottled appearance they are frequently softer and taste better.

One of my favorite types of plum is the so-called Italian prune or plum, available from the end of July through the end of September. These plums are reasonably priced and very good, but you have to catch them just right. In the beginning of the season they are often too hard and not edible. They also may quite rapidly become brown and rotten on the inside around the pit. For good taste, when fresh or in pies, the fruit should have golden yellow flesh without any spoilage around the pit and they should come off the pit easily without adherence.

Plums that are very longitudinal and have green flesh that clings to the pit are inferior. Italian prunes of high quality are easier to find in Europe (particularly Germany, Switzerland, Hungary, Austria, Belgium and other countries) than in the U.S., and unfortunately are not exported from these countries.

However, diligent shoppers in the U.S. will find them and be rewarded with excellent taste. These plums are used for plum pies—very popular throughout Central Europe.

Greengages are also plums but can be hard to find. Don't buy them unless they are ripe and soft. The skin is green, but when they are ripe they may have a yellow or orange tinge and they can be delicious. Europe has a small type of greengage which can be very sweet and flavourful.

Emperor and Empress plums arrive later in the season. They are longitudinally shaped and larger than the prune plum. They can be excellent when ripe, but often the pit is cracked and pieces spread through the fruit posing a danger to the teeth and to the throat when swallowed by accident.

Among other plums at the stores are Dinosaur plums. All need optimum ripeness for pleasurable eating. Certain plum varieties are hybrids with apricots and other fruits.

Plums available on the European continent include the very flavorful but small "Mirabelle", and the somewhat sour purple "Damson" plum of England. It is used in making preserves and has some similarities with the U.S. Beach plum. The Mirabelle, in addition to its consumption as fresh fruit, is used in liquors and for jams.

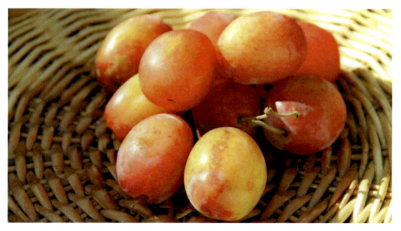

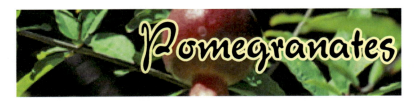

Pomegranates

This is a tropical fruit widely used in Asia, Egypt and other Near East countries. It has a history of culinary and medical applications. The fruit contains many black seeds and a pink to deep red gelatinous material around the seeds that is the edible portion. For eating pomegranates, they have to be peeled.

A pomegranate should have a red color, a firm smooth skin and a large size so that there is enough gelatinous material around the seeds to make it worth eating.

The easiest way to consume pomegranate is in the form of juice. In addition to valuable vitamins and minerals the juice contains antioxidants and physiologically active components that have been reported to be beneficial for immunity and heart function. Other health benefits have also been reported.

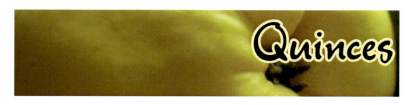

Quinces

The quince is related to both apples and pears and is yellow. Turkey is the country with the highest production of quince, but it is common in both the Balkan region and the Middle East.

The history of the quince goes back many centuries and is mentioned in classical Greek literature. It is even possible that the fruit referred to in the Garden of Eden was quince and not apple.

The quince is mostly eaten not as a fresh fruit, but only after cooking because it is too hard and sour. However, upon boiling the quince turns sweeter and the color of the flesh becomes pink. The most frequent times that I have come across quince are in jams and jellies eaten with cheese. After peeling they can also be used for roasting, baking, or stewing, usually as a minor additive to other foods.

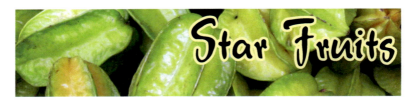

Star Fruits

In recent years star fruit, also called *carambola*, has increased in popularity in the United States. It has been grown for centuries in parts of Asia and now is grown also in Puerto Rico, Hawaii and Florida. Star fruit is most palatable when ripe, indicated by a yellowish green glossy color.

Caution! While Star Fruit is rich in vitamin C and antioxidants, it can also have negative effects on health: it contains oxalic acid, which can be a contributor to kidney stones and renal disease. It also causes drug interactions, particularly with statins (such as Lipitor) and with diazepines (such as Valium).

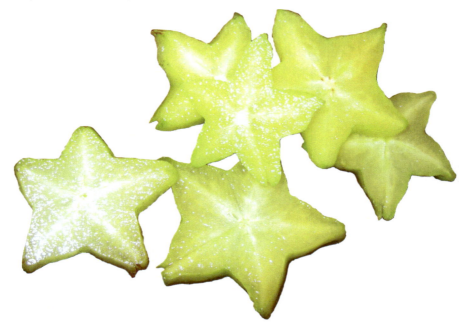

BERRY FRUITS

The consumption of berries has greatly increased in recent years.

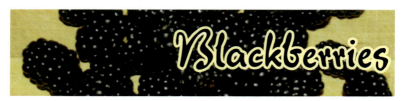

Blackberries

One of the greatest contributors to brambles is the blackberry bush. They catch your fabric when you get anywhere near and you learn to watch out when you live in the temperate climate where they grow wild. Blackberries grow in thickets at the edge of the forest and also in hedgerows. The berries ripen July to September and they are a delicious treat when you hike in areas where they grow. However, at times they are stunted and dried out. This I have never seen with the commercially grown berries that are being bred to get larger and sweeter. Though domesticated comparatively recently, you see blackberries more and more at the store, at the market, and at the table.

Blackberries are very high in antioxidants and are a good source of Vitamin C. When buying them, just like with other berries, you have to watch for mold—a sign that they have been picked under very moist conditions or too long ago. Their seeds are hard on the teeth and the digestion and probably should be avoided by people who have a tendency towards diverticulitis.

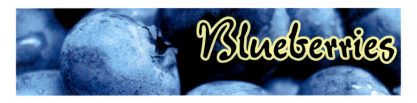

Blueberries

I know blueberries from picking them in the swamps and woods in the foothills of the Bavarian Alps, where I was born, and I will always remember the lovely and delicious blueberry pies my mother used to make. Having lived in the U.S. for the majority of my life, I have seen the development of this delicious, nutritious and healthy berry-fruit into the very important commercial crop it is today, particularly in New Jersey and Wisconsin.

Blueberry bushes come in three heights: low, medium and high. The low and medium bushes grow mainly in the wild and the high bushes in home gardens and in commercial berry farms, although they can occur in the wild where I have picked many in the Shawanguk Mountains. I have three high bush plants in my New Jersey garden now, but I never can harvest any berries because my avian and mammalian competitors get them before I do. The animals do not wait for optimum ripeness. As soon as the berries show a trace of blue, they are gone in a flash.

Blueberries are very healthful and full of antioxidants. The deeper the blue color the higher they score in tests for antioxidants. Blueberries are claimed to have medicinal properties, particularly as anticancer agents.

Commercially-grown American blueberries do not stain a tablecloth as much as those that are picked in the wild in Europe. The European wild berry has a very intense blue color produced by anthocyanins, which is the chemical name for the group of pigments that give these fruits and many other plants their color and which at the same time have antioxidant properties.

Cultivated blueberries are getting larger and larger and the season for availability gets longer and longer, as growers achieve further strain improvements. Blueberries are imported from South America during the off-season, so they are available almost year around, at a price.

When buying blueberries, the most important consideration is the absence of mold, which can be detected by appearance (white areas) and smell. Also they should not be dried out or wrinkled. Commercially dried blueberries are available as a snack for hikers.

Blueberry stains are very hard to remove from textiles, particularly if they are not fresh. The best is to work on removal right away with soap and hot water and a later hot machine wash usually finishes the job.

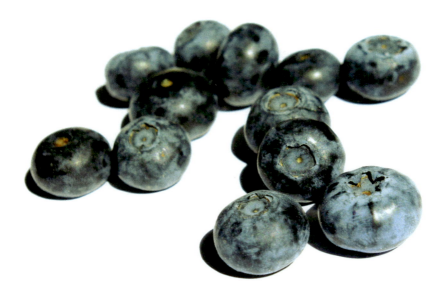

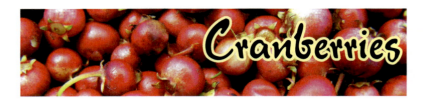

Cranberries

For Thanksgiving, Christmas, and New Years we usually eat cranberries in the form of compote to go with turkey. These red berries grow in swampy areas and are cultivated mainly in Wisconsin, New Jersey and Massachusetts.

Their bright red color tells you that they are full of the antioxidant anthocyanins, which as previously mentioned, are responsible for the colors of most fruits and flowers.

As true for other berries, these antioxidants may reduce the probability of getting cancer and heart disease. Cranberries also benefit patients with urinary infections and contain antimicrobial substances including benzoic acid.

They have a tangy taste, a mixture of sweet and acidic. In addition to their use in compote, they are frequent constituents of desserts, particularly baked goods such as cookies. Fresh cranberries are in the markets in the fall and can be stored fresh and frozen for use in the holiday season. When buying cranberries one should watch that they have good color, are plump and show no blemishes. Cranberry sauce (compote) is used year around with meat to add a sweet fruity taste. Cranberry juice is very available and healthy, and has a popular refreshing taste.

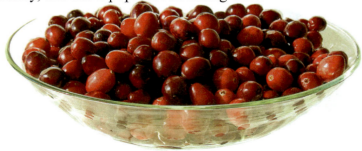

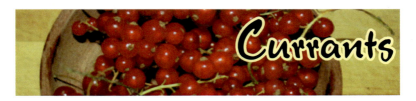

Currants

Currants come in red and white to cream-colored and black varieties, all having a slightly different but sweetish, acidic taste. They are widely grown and marketed in central and northern Europe and are now available for a short season in some U.S. markets. Redcurrants are the most popular; the black ones have a distinct taste.

Blackcurrants contain one of the greatest amounts of Vitamin C of any fruits.

Currants can be eaten fresh (usually sugar has to be added) or they are incorporated into desserts and are popular in the form of juices. Red and black currant juices are commercially bottled in Switzerland, Germany, and in some of the Scandinavian countries.

Currants grow on bushes similar to those of the gooseberry. These bushes usually are 1-3 feet high and can reach up to 6 feet in height.

Prior to the 1960s it was federally prohibited to grow currants or gooseberries in the United States because they can carry the white pine blister rust, which is very damaging to the white pine, an important tree for the wood industry. In 1966 this was changed and it is now up to the individual states whether these bushes may be grown. Their culture is permitted in Connecticut, New York State, and New Jersey but to date several other states have retained the ban.

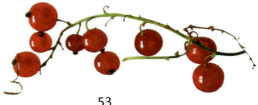

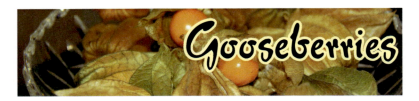

Gooseberries

Gooseberries have been available in the eastern U.S. markets for a comparatively short time, because of the same federal ban mentioned for currants. They are very popular throughout central and northern Europe and are making a comeback in the U.S. where the ban has been lifted.

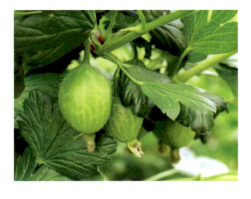

They grow well in home gardens on the eastern seaboard with red, yellow, and red/green mottled varieties. From my life in Europe I am well familiar with these varieties and others that are considerably larger; in England, Germany and the Scandinavian countries they are very popular and many larger varieties exist there. They are delicious when ripe but caution is needed to prevent them from getting overripe, mushy and off-taste. In addition to their consumption as the fresh berry, they are often used in desserts and for jams.

Gooseberries are round and have edible seeds and a sweet flavorful gelatinous mass clinging to the seeds. They have a hard skin when unripe but as the berry softens so does the skin. The skin is usually not eaten.

Ripeness is determined by squeezing them slightly and when they yield to the pressure it is usually the time of ripeness.

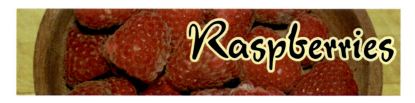

Raspberries

These are one of the most aromatic and delicious fruits; they can be picked wild in season, and cultivated to be available all year.

Beyond eating them fresh they are an absolute must for many desserts. Sugar enhances the raspberry flavor. Raspberries are used in jellies and praline fillings, juices and syrup; in addition a liqueur is made from raspberries. They are usually harvested as a copious crop in June or early July and depending on weather there is a skimpy second crop in late October or November. As a home garden crop they have to be protected from avian and mammalian predators.

They are a fragile fruit and have to be treated very carefully from harvest to consumption.

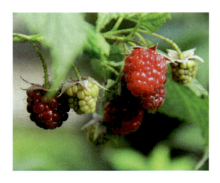

A white raspberry has been developed and sometimes it appears on store shelves, but I see no advantages in its flavor. There is a black raspberry which grows wild and is smaller and less juicy and there are several other edible relatives, but most are not cultivated.

In my childhood in Germany many raspberries were infected by little white worm-like insect larvae, but in the last 50 years they seem to been eradicated.

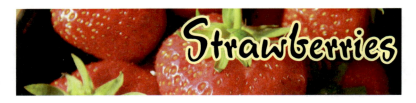

Strawberries

Aroma, flavor, texture and physical condition are determinants of quality for strawberries. Size is much overemphasized in advertisements. The best strawberry with optimum, melt-in-the-mouth flavor, is the one that is freshly picked in the backyard (if you have avoided damage from slugs and spoilage). In buying strawberries shipped from distant locations you have to give up something for getting fruit in good condition: a harder and more durable fruit for shipping has been developed by selection and plant breeding. Often you have to compromise on texture and ripeness; much of the fruit available is too firm and partially unripe, but you should not accept fruit of poor aroma and condition.

When purchasing berries you absolutely have to use your nose. By smelling at the openings of the box you can determine not only aroma but also whether any of the berries

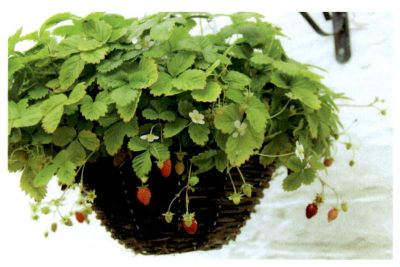

inside the container have become moldy. Particularly try to examine those at the bottom of the container.

Also look visually for any moldy berries and do not buy even if you see just one such berry, because other berries also have been infected and will mold within hours. The same rules apply to raspberries, blueberries, and blackberries. Do not buy moldy berries!

For strawberries the container they come in is also important. They should not be packed too tightly. Certain containers with tight wrapping, usually green in color, are in my opinion unfavorable. I have had berries from such containers that had a certain off flavor and since then I avoid them.

While strawberries usually just have one crop in late spring, ever-bearing berries exist that are usually much smaller but yield berries from spring to fall. There is a delicious wild strawberry that grows predominantly at the edge of the forest and is highly prized in restaurants and farm markets in Central and Northern Europe. It is very small but highly flavorful.

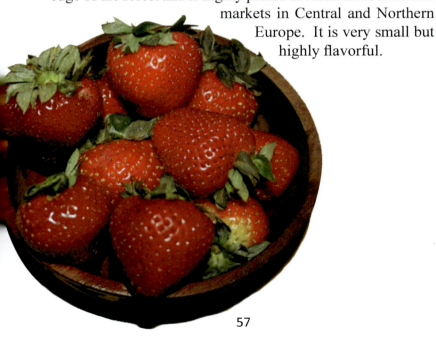

Chapter 2:
WHAT TO DO WITH THE FRUIT AFTER YOU GET IT HOME

When you get home from shopping you should have a plan for when and in what form you want to consume your fruit in order to eat it at optimum ripeness. The question is how to achieve this? Fruits can be divided into two groups according to their capability of ripening at home. The difference between these groups is that the ones that will ripen produce ethylene, the ripening hormone, while those that will not ripen do not produce ethylene. The ethylene producers are called climacteric while the non-ripening ones are non-climacteric. This subject will be dealt with further in a later section of the book.

Another decision is how the fruit should be cleaned and stored before consumption. There are three reasons for washing fruit: the removal of as much pesticide residue as possible, the removal of pathogenic microbes and the removal of soil and dirt.

Presence of pesticide and the harm caused by them has frequently been discussed in the general and scientific press as well as on TV. There have been panicky stories about their being the cause ailments from rheumatic diseases to arthritis, respiratory and other illnesses. According to the Environmental Working Group, 2010 lists presented in the Bergen Record on March 15, 2011, the produce with the highest amount of pesticide are peaches, strawberries, apples, blueberries, nectarines, cherries, and imported grapes. The fruits with least amount of pesticide are: avocado, pineapple, mango, kiwi, melons, and grapefruit.

The concerns about pesticides have elicited the development of orchards where methods are employed to grow fruits organically without use of chemicals, and now there are large sections in supermarkets selling organic produce. The USDA and FDA are government agencies that are our watchdogs to protect us from toxic and other contaminating agents in our food products.

There are other reasons for having concerns about eating unwashed fruit. Much produce is imported and it is physically impossible to test all batches, whether in the U.S. or abroad. Some handlers are responsible, but others may use shortcuts at the farm to save time and labor. And while questionable pesticide residues may be present only at non toxic amounts, combinations of pesticides may have different toxic effects and not all possible combinations have been adequately researched.

Another much more compelling reason, and one that few people think of, is the possible presence of pathogenic microbes. While most of our foods are heated before consumption or disinfected by pasteurization or other methods, this is not so with fruits, salads and some vegetables. Most fruit is washed at the farm, and the body's immune system incapacitates many potential pathogens, but there still occasionally occur viable pathogenic bacteria or protozoa on fruits. During the many years I have been a microbiologist I know of a few such cases: apples that had been dropped in a field contaminated by cow manure were subsequently used to make cider, and sickened many people with pathogenic E.coli; raspberries from South America contaminated by pathogenic protozoa that caused stomach upsets, and melons carrying salmonella. In 2011 there was a severe listeria epidemic from cantaloupe melons with many deaths. The cause of this epidemic has not yet been published. But these are only a few cases compared to the billions of shipments going out to consumers, though some incidences of food poisoning are never reported.

Wash your produce in plain water. Rinsing is often enough, but for some fruits a soak for 10-15 min in water is a good idea, followed by a simple rinse. For peaches, and other fruits with fuzzy skin, washing in hot water is useful and removes more pesticides; if done just under the tap there is no noticeable deterioration in quality. After washing, the fruit should be dried so that spoilage by molds is prevented or delayed. I always wash my fruit only just before consumption as the quality is preserved this way. Some fruits are very delicate and have to be washed with great care, particularly raspberries. I let them rest only for a couple of minutes in cold water and dry them briefly on a paper towel immediately before serving. Washing well is particularly important for preparing strawberries, as they grow near or on the soil, and also for grapes, as these may carry a considerable load of pesticide.

No washing or other method of cleaning, results in 100% removal of microbes or pesticides. In some fruits, microbes and/or chemicals can penetrate the skin and cannot be reached by water or other cleaning agents. For these possibilities we have to trust our ever-present immune system to protect us, without which we would be in jeopardy throughout life.

After purchase the desirable storage temperature depends on ripeness. Unripe climacteric fruit has to be kept at room temperature until ripe. Three particularly desirable taste sensations are connected with fruit: flavor, sweetness and refreshing qualities. Many fruits taste better when eaten not too cold; on the other hand fruits spoil easily and this is best prevented by chilling in the refrigerator. So a compromise is necessary, and personal preference should reign. I like most fruit refrigerated but apples, pears, nectarines, cherries, strawberries and raspberries appear to have more flavor when not so cold. This can be achieved by eating within hours after purchase or picking; otherwise to get the optimum flavor they have to be removed from the refrigerator for a while before consumption to get the optimum flavor. Bananas should not be refrigerated.

When making fruit salad, there are special problems. Peeled or cut fruits of several types blacken fast depending on specific variety. As mentioned previously, this is a biochemical process and caused by oxidation of compounds (phenolics) in the fruit; these, under the influence of oxygen from the air, are converted further by an enzyme to a darker polymer.

Fruits which darken rapidly include avocado, most kinds of apples, bananas, pears and peaches. This process is somewhat slowed by chilling. The darkening can be prevented by blanching (heating to kill the responsible enzymes), but then you no longer have the texture, flavor and appearance of fresh fruit. Lemon juice increases the acidity (lowers the pH) and also can be used to inhibit the enzyme responsible for the blackening. This is usually the preferred method of preventing this phenomenon. In some apples the enzymes responsible for this blackening have been removed by selective breeding such as with Red Delicious apples whose flesh hence can remain white for some time even when exposed to the air. Red Delicious is an apple used frequently in fruit baskets. In addition to its resistance to blackening it has very good keeping quality when being held at room temperature for some time.

Chapter 3:
NUTRITION AND HEALTH

The beneficial nutritional value of fruits is well-known and may be described and summed up as: low-calorie, high in soluble and insoluble fiber and rich in several of the essential vitamins and trace minerals.

Furthermore they have a beneficial effect on the digestion, combating constipation without being too laxative, and usually do not cause griping. For these reasons they are part of many reducing diets. Fruits are not nearly as high in sugar as many of the other desserts and thus are more freely permitted for people who must control their sugar intake because they are diabetic or for other reasons. Also due to their taste appeal fruits are palatable and accepted by patients who may be undernourished; often fruits are preferred over vegetables by children, and make it easier to provide them with a healthy diet.

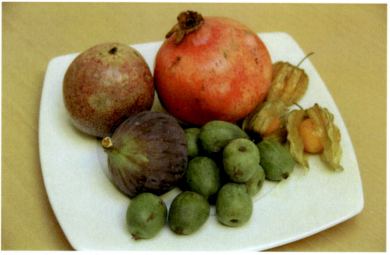

Fruit selection (clockwise from top left): passion fruit, pomegranate, Cape gooseberries, baby kiwis, fig.

Apart from their intrinsic properties, some fruits have special medicinal properties due to their particular constituents. As mentioned earlier in this book, both pineapple and papaya contain proteolytic enzymes. In the case of pineapple it is bromelain and in papaya it is papain. Both fruits are considered digestion promoters because of these proteolytic enzymes. Further, papain is used in a process to prevent beer from becoming cloudy due to protein hazes. Some fruits have constituents of their essential oil fraction, which are used in alternative medicine.

Antioxidants are trace constituents of fruit and they are very beneficial for human health. It is believed that oxidative processes caused by free radicals are harmful and have a role in cancer formation, heart disease, and aging. These oxygen-containing free radicals can be counteracted by antioxidants for which fruits are a major source. This is a chief reason why fruits are considered an important healthy food.

The group of agents to which belong Vitamin C, anthocyanins, biflavanoids, lutein, zeaxanthin, carotene and Vitamins A and E are mainly biochemical-reducing agents which combine with these free radicals and inactivate them. These antioxidants can be effective because they are very reactive, but this makes them also sensitive to environmental influences. They are diminished by storage, even in the refrigerator and they decay more rapidly at room or higher temperatures.

Almost all fruits have antioxidants, particularly prunes, all berry fruits, apples, cherries, oranges, red grapes, and raisins as well as many others.

I have observed that animals which prey on plants have a preference for flowers and colorful berries which leads me to believe that they have an instinct to eat the anthocyanin containing parts of the plants which have the most color (for instance, the flowers of lilies for deer and the heads of dandelions for rabbits).

Here I will describe the major and minor constituents.

Major Constituents

Fruits are made up of water, fiber, soluble carbohydrate, and a small amount of protein; with a few exceptions they contain almost no fat. The fiber has a soluble and an insoluble portion. The soluble fiber consists mainly of pectin, which is unique to plants. Pectin has an important function for human digestion. It binds fat and cholesterol and is reported to reduce heart disease. Both insoluble fiber and soluble fiber are beneficial for the digestion and ameliorate constipation. It also has been reported to bind fat; so this is not absorbed and it can prevent weight gain. Fiber gives the fruit its structure and turgor. There are other carbohydrates such as hemicelluloses, which are also part of soluble fiber. The insoluble fiber is mainly made up of cellulose. The high water content of fruit is a positive contributor. It makes fruits juicy, easy to swallow, thirst quenching, lower calorie, and very palatable.

Structure and composition of fruits is quite unique and makes them so desirable for human and animal consumption. This attraction for our competitors, the animals, insects and others who so often get ahead of us in harvesting them before we do, produces a need for pesticides and repellents. As discussed in the previous chapter there has been much concern in society about our ingestion of pesticides, because what is toxic for animals is also very likely toxic to man. We are to some extent protected from being sickened by the work of the Food and Drug Administration (FDA), whose job is to do just that. However there always will be some uncertainties about what happens when you consume these agents over your total life span and what happens if there is mutual reinforcement of toxicity, when several of these pesticides are consumed simultaneously or within a short time. It could also be that there might be interactions with medications. It appears however that the government agencies have done a good job in selecting permitted pesticides. The average life span of man is increasing and no conclusive evidence exists of severe health effects from pesticides in fruits when the application is at the permitted levels.

A whole new additional line of organic fruits has been developed which have been grown without pesticides. In some cases quality and taste of these organic fruits is better than that of regular ones. In other cases looks and quality are inferior. It is not easy to grow fruit organically on a commercial scale; one approach for avoiding pesticides has been the use of natural enemies of the pests such as predatory insects.

To grow 'organic' fruits, you have to grow all fruit-bearing crops without using chemicals; so apart from not using pesticides you must not apply chemical fertilizers or soil treatment materials. The whole method of agriculture has to be changed. This may entail a rotation of crops and the use of organic fertilizers such as manure or composted plants. For some consumers being able to purchase fruits without pesticide gives them peace of mind and eliminates their worry about chemicals, and particularly pesticides in their fruits even if they eat them without removing the skin. Peel contains high amounts of pectin and some of the valuable trace constituents about which we will talk later. Organic foods also give the farmer a chance to sell a premium product and thus achieve a higher price.

Another potentially promising method that would decrease the need for pesticides is being developed. This is genetic alteration of fruits to include genes that produce substances targeted against those insects or fungi that cause most crop loss in the particular fruit, and thus such fruit would have no need for pesticides.

Trace Constituents

Like all living beings, men and women require numerous biochemical substances to make life and health possible. Some of these necessary agents can be produced by our own metabolism, but others have to be supplied by nutrients, among them fruits. They may have been synthesized by the plant or concentrated from the environment. Many of the substances are needed only in trace quantities. A few of these trace minerals and vitamins will be discussed in more detail. There are many others that also are important but will not be dwelled on in this book. There are numerous tables published which give amounts of the trace constituents. Some of the values found differ widely. Of course this is to be expected, because these values depend on many factors, both genetic and environmental, the size and dry weight, maturity, ripeness, location on the tree, temperature exposed to, nutrients, compounds in the water the plant absorbs, moisture conditions during growth, the ratio of fruits to leaves and roots, etc. The possible factors are extremely varied. Values determined by scientists can be found on the internet and in books on nutrition.

The best known of the essential substances is Vitamin C, also called ascorbic acid. This substance is an anti-oxidant and is needed by man for the immune system and to prevent scurvy. The symptoms of scurvy are fatigue, sore and swollen gums, loose teeth and skin problems. If not treated by Vitamin C, it can lead to death. This disease, which often affected sailors on long trips when no fresh fruits were available, taught people the importance of Vitamin C in the form of lemon juice. Vitamin C is only produced by plants, and we have to continuously replenish this substance in our systems.

The fruits with the greatest amounts of Vitamin C are those shown in Table 4 in order of concentration:

Table 4:

Highest Amount of Vitamin C	
1. Black Currant	6. Orange
2. Blackberry	7. Papaya
3. Kiwi	8. Lemon
4. Strawberry	9. Lime
5. Kumquat	10. Grapefruit

All fruits have some Vitamin C. The highest Vitamin C concentration has been reported at 155-215 milligrams (mg) per 100 grams of blackcurrant, while the popular orange analyses at 45-55 mg per 100 grams. The daily requirement for Vitamin C is 90mg for men and 75 for women.

Vitamin A is another vitamin for which fruits are an important source. Table 5 gives a list of the fruits richest in vitamin A; however there are many other dietary sources of this vitamin such as leafy vegetables and dairy products. Carotene, which is plentiful in carrots, fulfils many of the same physiological functions as Vitamin A. The daily requirement for Vitamin A is 0.7-1 mg. Vitamin A is important for visual and muscular functions.

Table 5: Some fruits which have high Vitamin A content

High in Vitamin A
Grapefruit
Cantaloupe
Watermelon
Mango
Guava
Plum
Peach & Papaya
Nectarine
Orange

Fruits are a source for another important vitamin: Vitamin K. Humans have a minimum dietary requirement for Vitamin K of 2 mg/day. The fruit with highest reported amount of Vitamin K is kiwi followed by raspberry, avocado, and blackberry. This vitamin is important for bone structure and blood clotting. There are many other good dietary sources for this vitamin such as meat and vegetables. Fruits can only supply a small amount of minimum daily requirement. In addition to C, A and K almost all fruits contain smaller amounts of other vitamins.

Fruits are also rich in minerals; their high content of potassium and magnesium is particularly important.

Table 6: Fruits high in Potassium

POTASSIUM
Avocado
Guava
Kiwi
Banana
Papaya
Black Currants
Grapefruit
Pear
Grapes
Plum

The minimum requirement for potassium is 2000 mg/day. The avocado is reported to contribute 900-1000 mg of potassium per 100 grams of fruit and can supply a large portion of the minimum daily requirement.

Magnesium at a minimum daily requirement of about 400 mg a day is most abundant in raspberries of which 100 grams will supply one quarter of this requirement.

Table 7: Fruits high in Magnesium

MAGNESIUM
Avocado
Grapefruit
Guava
Kiwi
Pineapple
Raspberries
Strawberry
Watermelon

Fruits usually fulfill only part of the daily requirement of these minerals; other foods will fill the rest.

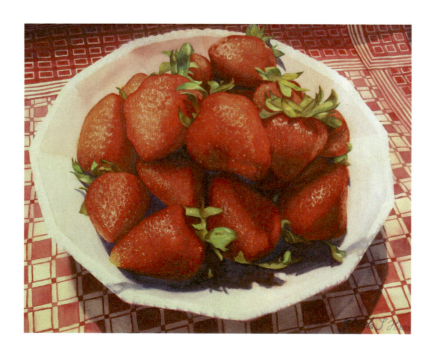

Chapter 4:
SOME ASPECTS OF FRUIT BIOCHEMISTRY AND THEIR IMPACT ON QUALITY

The Ripening Process

Fruit exists for the propagation of plants, containing the seeds for and continuation of existence of their kind and of their genes.

Their attraction and appeal is a lure for a wide range of animals of which mankind is just one. Their consumption by animals and by ourselves, helps the dissemination of seeds, and the resulting fruit species, over a wide area. The actual seed is a small part of the fruit; the outer shell is made up of the flesh and peel which have to be removed for the seeds to be able to find a good location in the soil and germinate successfully. The flesh of fruit can be removed by insects, by numerous animals, and also by microorganisms. This removal of the flesh should only occur if the seeds are ripe and can germinate. If seeds are unripe there will be no germination and they will die. To this end the whole fruit ripens at the same time as the seed.

As can be seen in apples and pears when they are ready to be eaten, the pips in the core have turned black and are ready to sprout. Plant hormones are involved in the ripening process. The most important of these hormones is ethylene, a gas produced by plants from metabolizing the amino acid methionine. Ethylene increases the enzymes amylase and pectinase. Amylase hydrolyzes the starch to produce sugars and pectinase decreases the molecular weight of pectin and thus the hardness of the fruit. Other enzymes degrade and decolorize the green pigment chlorophyll and the fruits may change their color to blue, yellow, orange, and red.

Ethylene can be applied to speed up ripening of unripe fruit. Some fruits are shipped unripe and ripened by addition of ethylene before they are sold. Bananas and some other fruits produce appreciable ethylene themselves and a ripe banana can help a green banana to ripen more rapidly, particularly if they are held jointly in a paper bag. Several enzymes are involved in the production of ethylene. There are agents that delay ripening so that the unripe fruit is less vulnerable to bruising and spoilage in the shipping process. This fruit subsequently can be ripened with ethylene in the warehouse before sale. One of the potential ripening inhibitors is methyl cyclopropene.

The process of ripening with ethylene is only successful when the fruit has been picked not too unripe. I tried to ripen a honeydew melon in a paper bag together with bananas. While several bananas were used one after the other and ripened in the paper bag, the melon stayed stubbornly hard and was finally cut after about 3 months storage. It had very little aroma and still somewhat hard, though edible.

The length of time it takes for a given fruit to ripen in nature is genetically determined as well as influenced by the weather. For optimum chances of reproduction it must coincide with the time most favorable for the seeds to germinate. Also the right birds and animals should be present to ensure wide dissemination.

As mentioned, fruits can be divided into climacteric and non-climacteric. In an earlier section pears were identified as a climacteric fruit. Climacteric fruits are capable of generating ethylene to allow them to ripen after harvest. In contrast, non-climacteric fruits do not ripen after picking and are not affected by ethylene. The table below is taken from the Food and Agriculture Organization (FAO) Corporate

Document Repository, Manual for the preparation and sale of fruits and vegetables, PDF version.

Table: 8: Climacteric vs. Non-climacteric Fruits

NON-CLIMACTERIC	CLIMACTERIC
Must be purchased ripe	Will ripen further if desired, will not ripen if abused during packing or storage
Blackberries	Apples
Blueberries	Apricots
Cherries	Avocados
Grapes	Bananas
Grapefruits	Figs
Lemons	Guavas
Limes	Kiwi fruits
Oranges	Mangoes
Pomegranates	Melons
Raspberries	Nectarines
Strawberries	Papayas
	Passion fruits
	Peaches
	Pears
	Plantains
	Plums

RECIPES FROM AROUND THE WORLD

As fruits are used in different ways by different cultures and nations, I have tried to collect a few recipes popular in specific countries. Before reading this section, it must be realized by the reader that my selection is very haphazard. I have taken recipes with which I am familiar or where I have friends who gave me such a recipe. Also, the inclusion of a particular recipe by no means indicates that this is the only version or even the most popular fruit dish in any country. There are many regional differences and different opinions by people who prepare, cook or consume a particular item. Most of the recipes can also be found in cookbooks or on the Internet and in no way can they be considered proprietary to the author.

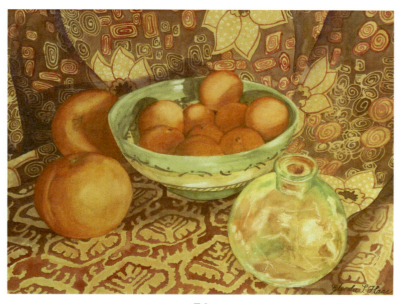

ASIA

ARMENIA

Date Cookies

Ingredients for dough:

4 cups flour

1 cup of cream of wheat (Farina)

1 cup butter (2 sticks)

¼ cup corn oil

¾ cup milk

2 teaspoons baking powder

¼ cup sugar

1 egg (to be used as a glaze)

½ teaspoon ground Mahlab (Middle Eastern spice) (optional)

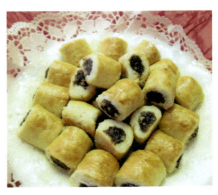

Ingredients for date filling:

1 ½ lbs. dates

3 tablespoons corn oil

3 tablespoons butter

½ teaspoon ground cinnamon

1 cup walnuts

Preparation of dough:

    Mix flour, baking powder, and cream of wheat together. Melt the butter on low heat and add milk. Add butter mixture, along with the corn oil, to the flour mixture. Mix all together and work by hand into soft dough. Afterwards, divide the dough into eight equal, separate portions.

Preparation of filling:

Mash the dates. Warm the butter on low heat. Grind the walnuts in a nut grinder. Mix the mashed dates, corn oil, and melted butter in a sauté pan on very low heat until dates become paste-like. Stir often to prevent dates from sticking to pan. Add the ground walnuts and cinnamon to the softened date mixture. Stir all together thoroughly. Remove from heat and allow to cool.

Preparation of cookie:

With rolling pin, flatten one of the eight portions of dough to a 4" wide x 14" long sheet. Take portion of date filling and roll by hand into a 14" long x 3/4" wide cylinder-like shape. Place onto edge of flattened dough. Roll the dough over the date filling as if making a "cigar-like" form, until date filling is completely covered and there is no more flattened dough to roll over it. Place onto a sheet of parchment paper, atop a 17" x 12" cookie tray. Repeat same for the remaining seven portions of dough and date filling. You will now have eight "cigar-like" rolls on the tray.

Beat the egg. Brush the egg onto the top of all eight rolls. Finally, cut the rolls width-wise into 1" pieces. This will yield approximately 80 individual cookies in total. Bake in oven at 375°F for 25-30 minutes until top of cookies turn a light, golden brown. Remove from oven and let cool for 30 minutes.

Contributed by: Shakeh Barsoumian

INDIA

Chikoo (Mamaey Sapote) Halwa (Pudding):

Ingredients:

6 Chikoos (can be obtained in the US in Indian and South American grocery stores)

½ cup milk

¼ cup sugar

⅔ cup khoya (aka reduced milk or dried milk, readily available in Indian grocery stores)

2-3 drops vanilla essence

1 tablespoon ghee (clarified butter, readily available in Indian grocery stores)

Preparation:

Peel and mash the chickoos. Add milk to the mashed chickoos in a heavy saucepan and boil. When slightly thick, add khoya and cook while stirring continuously. Add sugar and ghee. Cook on low heat and stir until ghee oozes. Garnish with almonds or walnuts when served.

Several sources contributed for this recipe.

IRAN

Date Cakes

Ingredients:

- 3 cups pitted dates
- 1 cup coarsely chopped walnuts
- For dough:
- 1 cup unsalted butter
- 1 ½ cups sifted all-purpose flour
- ½ cup confectioners' sugar
- 1 teaspoon ground cinnamon
- ½ teaspoon ground cardamom
- 1 cup ground unsalted pistachios or shredded coconut for decoration

Makes 15 pieces
Preparation time: 30 minutes
Cooking time: 20 minutes

Preparation:

In a skillet, toast the walnuts over medium heat for 5 minutes. Set aside and allow to cool.

Place a few walnut pieces inside each date.

Arrange the dates, packed next to each other, in a flat 9-inch serving dish.

In a large deep skillet, fry the flour in butter over high heat, stirring constantly for about 15 to 20 minutes, until the mixture is a golden caramel color.

Spread the hot dough over the dates, and pack and smooth it well with the back of a spoon to create an even surface.

Meanwhile, combine the cinnamon, confectioner's sugar, and cardamom and sprinkle evenly over the cake.

Sprinkle with 1 cup ground pistachios or shredded coconut evenly all over the surface. Allow to cool.

Cut in small square-shaped pieces. Carefully arrange these on serving platter, or serve on the same plate.

This recipe is obtained from New Food of Life, A Book of Ancient Persian and Modern Iranian Cooking and Ceremonies.

CHILE

Apple and Quince Flan Caramel

Ingredients:

4 large apples, peeled, cored, and finely diced

1 quince, peeled, cored, and finely diced

3 to 4 ripe apricots or 1 guava or 2 peaches or 1/2 cup berries

½ cup plus 3 tablespoons water

1 ½ cups of sugar

2 tablespoons butter, at room temperature

1 teaspoon vanilla extract

3 eggs, separated

½ cup plain cookies, crushed to a fine powder with a rolling pin

Pinch of salt

Preparation:

Place the apples and quince in a large saucepan with ½ cup of water; bring to a boil. Reduce the heat and cook covered, stirring occasionally, until the fruit is very soft (10 to 15 minutes). Add ¼ cup of the sugar and cook, stirring constantly with a wooden spoon, over medium heat to reduce the liquid slightly (about 2 minutes). Set aside.

In a small bowl, whisk the butter with ¼ cup of the sugar until fluffy. Add the vanilla and whisk in the egg yolks, one at a time. Add the cookies. Stir the mixture into the fruit and combine well. Let cool.

Preheat the oven to 375°F.

Meanwhile, to prepare the caramel, combine the remaining 1 cup of sugar and 3 tablespoons of water in a heavy saucepan. Cook over high heat, stirring until the sugar is dissolved. Cook, without stirring, until the syrup caramelizes and turns a medium-dark amber, about 4 minutes. To stop the cooking, immerse the bottom of the pan into cold water. Divide the caramel quickly among 1-cup custard cups, or ramekins, swirling the cups to evenly coat the bottoms. Set aside.

Beat the egg whites with the salt in a medium size bowl until stiff but not dry.

Add one third of the beaten egg whites to the fruit mixture and mix well. Gently fold in the remaining whites. Divide the mixture evenly into the caramel-coated cups.

Place the ramekins (small glazed ceramic baking bowl) in a roasting pan and add enough hot water to come halfway up the sides of the pan. Bake in the center of the oven 35 to 40 minutes or until the custard is set. Remove the ramekins from the water bath and let sit about 15 minutes before unmolding. Serve warm, lukewarm, or chilled.

Contributed by: Nano Mardones

CUBA

Cascos de Guayaba:

Ingredients:

2 lbs fresh guavas

3 cups of water

3 cups of sugar

1 medium lime

4 ½ cups water

Preparation:

Peel the guavas and cut them into halves. Carefully remove the seeds and all of the flesh with a spoon. Reserve flesh for another use. Place the remaining hard skins in a large pot. Add water and boil for approximately one hour, until the shells are tender. Remove the boiled shells and set aside. Measure about 3 cups of the water that was used for boiling. Discard the remainder. Place the 3 cups of water back into the cooking pot and add the sugar and lime juice. Stir until dissolved. Add the cooked guava shells and leave, uncovered, for about 40-45 minutes, or until the syrup is thick and the guava shells tender enough to fold into themselves. You may then serve, accompanied with white or cream cheese, if desired.

Contributed by: Rudolph Milian

CZECH REPUBLIC – MORAVIA

Peach Cake

Ingredients:

1 ¾ cup flour

1 ½ teaspoon baking powder

½ cup butter (1 stick)

1 cup sugar

4 eggs

Grated peel of one lemon

4 tablespoons cream or milk

8 medium-sized peaches, peeled and sliced

Preparation:

In a small bowl, mix flour and baking powder thoroughly and set aside. In a larger bowl, cream butter until light and fluffy. Add sugar gradually while mixing it thoroughly. Beat in eggs, one at a time, and mix well. Add lemon peel.

Add flour to mixture, alternating with cream or milk. Spread batter in buttered coffee cake pan and cover dough with sliced peaches. Bake at 350° F for one hour.

Peaches can be substituted with apricots, blueberries, or apples.

Contributed by: Elizabeth Demarest

ENGLAND

Gooseberry Fool

Ingredients:

1 lb gooseberries

½ cup sugar

2 pints heavy cream (4 cups)

A little water

Preparation:

Cook the gooseberries in just enough water to stop them sticking to the pan. Add sugar to taste, then, push through a sieve. Whip the cream until it will stand in peaks, then blend the sieved gooseberries with the cream. Chill.

Contributed by: Eileen Barbour

Summer Pudding

Ingredients:

6 or 7 slices of white bread

2 lbs summer fruits such as, raspberries, red currants, blueberries, and black currants

4 tablespoons of white sugar

Preparation:

You need a 4-cup pudding bowl and a saucer that fits inside the rim.

Line the pudding bowl with slices of bread.

Rinse the prepared fruit and put it in a pan with 2 tablespoons of water and the sugar. Bring to the boil and simmer gently for 10 minutes, making sure it does not stick or burn.

Pour the mixture carefully into the lined bowl almost to the top. Cover with additional slices of bread. Put the saucer on the bread and put a small weight on the saucer. Put the bowl in the fridge overnight.

To serve, turn the pudding out onto a shallow bowl and cut into slices. Serve with yogurt or whipped cream, if desired.

Contributed by: Charlotte Morgan

Very Easy Trifle

Ingredients:

1 packet of trifle sponges or Madeira cake

1 can of mandarin orange segments

1 jar of raspberry or strawberry jam

5 cups fresh vanilla custard

1 pint whipping cream (about 1 cup)

Fresh strawberries or raspberries

Preparation:

Put a layer of sponge cake at the bottom of a large glass bowl.

Strain the mandarins and pour the juice over the sponges. You can add some orange or almond liqueur to the juice before you pour if you like.

Spread a layer of jam over the sponges.

Pour the vanilla custard over the jam.

Whip the cream until it is stiff and spread it over the custard.

Decorate with the drained mandarin segments and some fresh raspberries or strawberries (depending on the jam).

Contributed by: Charlotte Morgan

FRANCE

Pear Helene

Ingredients:

1 cup white wine

4 tablespoons sugar

½ tablespoon grated lemon peel

½ of a vanilla bean

3 ripe pears

½ cup cream

1 tablespoon honey

4 ounces (about ½ cup) bitter-sweet chocolate

5 cups (approximately) vanilla ice cream

⅓ cup chopped almonds

Preparation:

To poach the pears, place the wine into a pan with sugar and lemon peel. Add ¼ section of the vanilla bean, and bring to a boil. As soon as it boils, reduce the heat to medium.

Meanwhile, peel and half the pears. The stems may be removed or left on for decoration. Carefully remove seeds and core. Add the pears to the wine and cook over medium heat until glassy looking, about 20 minutes. Turn the pears once during the process. The cooked pears should still be firm enough to hold together. Leave the pears to cool in the wine syrup.

In a small pan, pour the cream, honey, and the other ¼ section of vanilla bean. Bring to a boil, then remove from heat. At the same time, melt the chocolate in a double boiler. Remove the vanilla bean from the cream mixture and fold the cream into the chocolate.

Remove the pears from the syrup and let drain on a paper towel. Prepare six individual bowls of ice cream and place a sliced pear half on each mound of ice cream. Divide the chocolate sauce between the portions and sprinkle with chopped almonds. Serve immediately.

Contributed by: Cornelia Muggenthaler

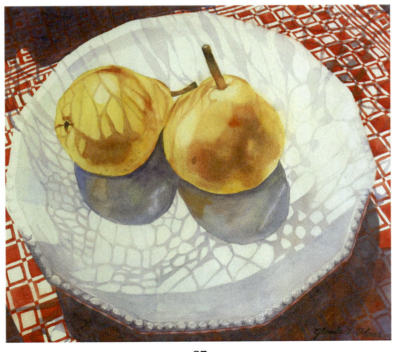

GERMANY

Rote Grütze (Red Fruit Dessert)

This refreshing summer pudding has as many variations as there are cooks, as changes can be made to reflect available fruits. The standard tradition calls for two sweet fruits, such as raspberries and strawberries, and two sour fruits, such as sour cherries and red currants. Since currants are not widely available in the U.S., cranberry juice makes an acceptable substitute. If two sweet fruits are not available, you may use double the quantity of one sweet fruit, and so on. Use the following as a general guide, but do not be afraid to substitute or experiment.

Ingredients:

½ lb. raspberries

½ lb. strawberries, chopped

½ lb. sour cherries, halved and pitted

½ lb. red currants

½ cup sugar

½ cup cornstarch

Whipped cream or vanilla sauce

Preparation:

Wash fruit and place in a large saucepan. Add about a quart of water and bring to a boil, uncovered. Continue to boil until the fruit has begun to fall apart.

Meanwhile, combine the cornstarch with 1 cup of water to make a smooth, thin paste. Add the corstarch to the boiling fruit and whisk it vigorously. Reduce the heat and cook, stirring constantly, for 3 to 5 minutes, or until mixture has thickened. It should appear translucent, rather than milky.

Because the Rote Grütze needs to cool completely before it will gel, make it well in advance. It can either cool at room temperature or in the refrigerator. Serve with whipped cream or vanilla sauce.

Contributed by: Renate Rattenhuber

GREECE

Yogurt with Fruit

Dairy and fruit is a winning combination consumed and loved in many countries. Ice cream, whipped cream, yogurt, and fine cheeses are all popular partners for a wide variety of fruits.

In Greece, whose yogurt is justifiably famous, honey is frequently added to the mixture. In one recipe for Yogurt Parfait, strained fat-free yogurt is mixed one to one with whole milk. Bread crusts from soft white bread are added, as well as lemon juice and honey or sugar to taste. After mixing the yogurt, sliced strawberries, blueberries, or peaches are added.

Contributed by: Dr. John S. Pantazopoulos

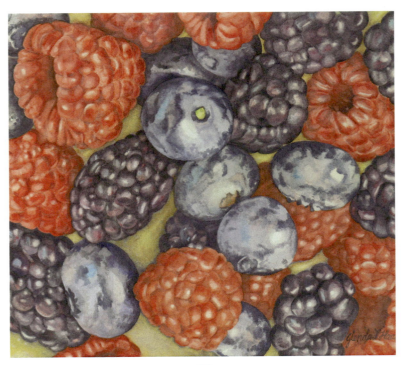

IRELAND

Apple Barley Pudding

Ingredients:

4 tablespoons Pearl Barley

3 tablespoons sugar

1 ½ lbs. apples, peeled, cored, and sliced

1 cup heavy cream

1 tablespoon lemon juice

Preparation:

Boil the barley in water and add the apples. Cook until both begin to soften. Drain and blend the mixture in a blender or sieve. Return the mixture to the cooking pot and bring to a boil again. Allow to cool and then chill. Top with cream when serving. Makes 4 servings.

ITALY

Crema Fredda di Limone e Lime
(Iced Lemon Cream)

Ingredients:

⅓ cup sugar

1 ⅓ cup cream

Flesh of 1 small lemon and its juice

Flesh of lime and its juice

2 teaspoons Marsala or Port wine (optional)

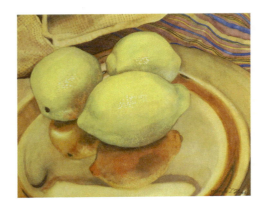

A few lime and lemon peel sprinkles

Preparation:

Mix the fruit, juice, sugar, and wine, if using, in a large bowl or blender container. Add the cream. Beat with an electric mixer or blender until the cream has thickened.

Pour into 6 serving cups or glasses, sprinkle with lemon peel, and refrigerate for at least 2 hours.

Serve with nice cookies. Almond crescents are recommended by the author.

Contributed by: Cornelia Muggenthaler

JAMAICA

Banana Cake

Ingredients for cake:

½ cup butter (1 stick)

1 cup of sugar

2 eggs

3 ripe bananas, peeled and mashed

2 cups sifted flour

1 teaspoon baking soda

½ teaspoon nutmeg powder

½ cup chopped cashew nuts

For topping:

4 egg whites

1 cup sugar

2 tablespoons light rum

Preparation:

For Cake

Cream butter and sugar. Beat in each egg one at a time. Add flour, soda, and nutmeg.

Add cashew nuts and bake at 350°F for about 50 minutes or until the knife comes out clean when put in the cake. Bake in an 8" greased cake pan.

For Topping

Beat egg whites gradually and add rum and sugar. Beat until the mixture holds a peak. Spread on cake.

Contributed by: Joan Benjamin.

MEXICO

Guacamole

Ingredients:

1 large avocado (If large avocado is not available, use 2 or 3 medium sized. The avocado needs to be ripe, but not too soft to the touch)

½ white onion

1 or 2 green chilies Serrano*

1 medium tomato

Several sprigs of fresh cilantro

1 tablespoon juice of fresh lime

Salt and pepper to taste

Preparation:

Peel, and cube the avocado. Cut white onion into very small pieces. Wash and seed the chilies; chop into small pieces. Wash, dry the cilantro and chop into small pieces; discard the stems. Cut tomato into small pieces. Mash the avocado with fork. Add the other ingredients and mix.

If making ahead of time, place the pit of the avocado into the guacamole, cover and refrigerate. The pit slows the blackening process. The pit may be removed when serving or left for decorative purposes. Serves 4

If you would like to make it spicier & hot, increase the chilies.

This recipe comes from Chef Pedro Cruz Morales, Restaurante Wala Wala, Avenida Juarez Esquna con Paredes, No. 183, San Blas, Nayarit, Mexico. Phone: 323 825 0863

Contributed by: Mike Green

PANAMA

Gazpacho

Ingredients:

5 lbs of ripe tomatoes (diced)

5 cloves garlic

Take out the mid core of a pineapple and peel. Then add about 1/8 of the whole pineapple

2 medium onions

2 red and 1 green bell pepper

1/8 of a medium sized melon

Add vinaigrette (¼ cup of cider vinegar to ¾ cup of olive oil)

Salt to taste

Preparation:

Fill a blender with 10% ice and add all the above ingredients. Blend until smooth and filter through a large colander to eliminate extra fiber.

Serve cool and fresh.

Contributed by Enrique Guardia, Panama.

POLAND

Pierogies with Blueberries

Ingredients:

For Dough:
- 1 egg yolk (slightly beaten)
- ½ cup lukewarm water
- 1 ½ teaspoon olive oil
- 2 cups sifted all-purpose flour
- ½ teaspoon salt

For Filling:
- 1 lb. blueberries
- 1 tablespoon sugar
- 1 teaspoon cinnamon powder

Optional Topping:
- 2 tablespoons sour cream
- 1 tablespoon sugar or melted butter

Preparation:

Whip olive oil with salt, egg yolk, and water. Beat in flour, a little at a time, to form stiff dough that does not stick to hands. Move dough to a large well floured cutting board and knead a few minutes until smooth. Cover with a bowl and allow to stand at room temperature for about 1 hour. This ripens the dough, making it easier to roll.

To prepare filling, mix blueberries, sugar and cinnamon in a large bowl.

Take a handful of dough and roll out into a thin rectangle. Cut out circles that are 3-4 inches in diameter. Place half a tablespoon of blueberry filling on each circle and fold sides together to create a semi-circle shape, pinching together edges to seal. Then, fill a large deep pot ¾ of the way with water, and bring to a boil. When boiling, add the raw pierogies and cook for about 12 minutes. They will float to the top when done. Once cooked, blanch them thoroughly with cold water and place in single layers on a flat platter. If you would like, you may pour your sour cream mixture or melted butter as a topping. This will make approximately 28-30 pierogies.

Contributed by: Teresa Cyburt

SLOVAKIA

Potato dumplings filled with Red Currant (or Plums or Apricots)

Ingredients:

1 lb. potatoes	*For Topping:*
1 cup all-purpose flour	½ cup butter (1 stick)
1 egg	¼ teaspoon cinnamon
1 cup red currants	⅓ cup ground walnuts
½ cup sugar	1 cup bread crumbs
	¼ cup sugar

Makes 40 portions.
60 minutes preparation time.
30 minutes additional time

Preparation:

Boil the potatoes with their skin and afterwards, peel the skin off.

Mash the potatoes, then add eggs, salt, and the flour and make a dough. Roll the dough out into 6-8 mm thick and make squares. Put some sugar and red currant into each square. Fold each square in half and seal edges. Fill a pot with water and some salt and bring water to boil. Add small batches of dumplings into the boiling water and wait until they rise to the top.

Meanwhile, brown the bread crumbs in butter. Add sugar and cinnamon sugar to this and brown together.

At the end, remove the dumplings and place them in a dish and cover with browned bread crumbs. Add a little bit of butter and walnuts on top.

Contributed by: Dr. Ivica Labuda

UNITED STATES OF AMERICA

Apple Pie:

Ingredients:

6-7 cups sliced, peeled Granny Smith apples

¾ cup sugar

¼ cup brown sugar

2 tablespoons all purpose flour

¾ teaspoon cinnamon

¾ teaspoon salt

⅛ teaspoon nutmeg

1 tablespoon lemon juice

Preparation:

Pre-heat the oven to 425°F. In a large bowl, combine all ingredients, tossing slightly. Spoon into frozen 9" pie shell. Dab with butter. Use a second frozen pie shell to cover top and crimp together the edges to make one. Slit the top pie shell in several places. Sprinkle lightly with cinnamon. Bake at 425°F for 40-45 minutes until golden brown.

Contributed by: Karen Eck

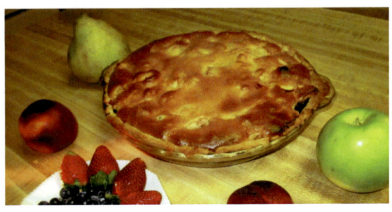

Poppy Seed Strawberry Shortcake:

Ingredients:

For Cake
- 2 ½ cups all purpose flour
- ¼ cup sugar
- 2 ½ tablespoons poppy seeds
- 3 ¼ tablespoons baking powder
- ½ teaspoon salt
- 4 ounces (1 stick) unsalted butter, cut into pieces
- 1 cup cream

For Filling
- 3 cups sliced strawberries
- 2 ¼ cups heavy whipping cream
- 1 teaspoon vanilla extract
- 1 ½ tablespoons sugar

To Assemble
- 3 tablespoons butter, softened
- 2 tablespoons powdered (10X) sugar

Preparation:

For Cake

Combine all the ingredients except cream in bowl of electric mixer. Mix on low speed until butter is the size of small peas. Slowly add cream and mix just until the dough comes together and forms a ball.

On a lightly floured surface, roll out the dough and cut into 3 inches circles. Brush the tops with 1 tablespoon of cream and sprinkle with 2 tablespoons of sugar.

Bake for 20 to 25 minutes at 350°F until golden brown.

For Filling

Combine all ingredients (except strawberries) in a bowl and beat until cream hold its shape.

To assemble, combine butter and sugar. Split the shortcakes in half and spread each half with sweetened butter. Place some strawberries and cream on the bottom half of each shortcake and top with the second half. Add more whipped cream, as desired. Serves 6

Contributed by: Glenda Haas

Appendix 1: METHODS FOR PRESERVING FRESH FRUIT

Anyone who has been shopping for several years will have observed that the time span of availability of specific fruits has increased continuously. Much of this is due to the wide spectrum of countries from which the fruits are imported and this importation allows prices to be close to those charged during the local season. To accomplish this is an amazing feat of modern technology.

As we all know, fruits are perishable to a greater or lesser extent and they are most perishable when picked ripe and at the peak of their palatability. Strawberries and raspberries deteriorate very rapidly when not refrigerated, even in a few hours. Apples and citrus and some other fruits are at the other end of the spectrum and can be kept at room temperature for an appreciable time; but even these more hardy fruits spoil eventually.

Unripe fruit can be ripened by holding for one or two days in a paper bag. A gunny sack or burlap bag will also work for this purpose. This is only useful for climacteric fruits which respond to ethylene. In the bag, the ethylene is closely held to the unripe fruit and this speeds ripening. Ripening can be speeded up even more by placing a high ethylene producer, such as bananas or apples, into the bag with the fruit you wish to ripen in a hurry. But you have to be careful you do not overshoot when you add a banana to an unripe peach, nectarine, or avocado in a paper bag so you do not end up with a mushy and unappetizing fruit. The paper bag procedure has been recommended for bananas, cranberries, kiwis, pears, avocados, sapotes, nectarines, peaches, and possibly melons and pineapples among others.

I do not use the paper bag method for my own fruit as it is so easy to leave it too long. I ripen my fruit on the counter at room temperature and when ripe transfer it into the refrigerator. Refrigeration is right for ripe apples, all berries, cherries, grapes, kiwis, melons, pears, persimmons, pomegranates, apricots, peaches, nectarines, and plums.

Prolonged storage of fruit at good quality is made possible by four technologies: refrigeration, the breeding of fruit varieties with less fragile texture and better keeping quality, adjustment in the atmosphere of storage (controlled atmosphere storage), the gentle transportation and packaging to avoid bruising. Rapid refrigeration is achieved by forcing refrigerated cold air through the containers. The aim is to cool the fruit to a temperature of 32°F (0°C) (but not lower to avoid freezing) within one hour of harvest and store under high humidity conditions. The cold temperature greatly slows down the ripening and spoilage. For apples this keeps the fruits in good condition for about four months. For longer storage the atmosphere is altered to lower oxygen (2.5%) and higher carbon dioxide (5%). These values are varied depending on which fruit you are preserving. The major crops using controlled atmosphere for storage are apples, pears, and kiwi. For strawberries, the atmosphere is adjusted during transportation depending on the distance the fruit has to travel and the time needed to get to the destination. The adjustment is again an increase in carbon dioxide and lowered oxygen. The increase in carbon dioxide has several beneficial effects. It retards ripening and kills many insect pests that are lurking in the fruits (coddling moths in apples, etc.), and it inhibits fungi and many bacteria, but a too high carbon dioxide level produces browning of the fruit and unfavorable changes in texture and flavor. Refrigerated trucks and special padding of the fruit reduce damage and, of course, shipment by air makes many of the described procedures unnecessary.

This technology has made it possible to eat cherries shipped from Chile in January and strawberries all year round. It also helps U.S. exports; for instance when visiting Japan I was greeted at the store by cherries in excellent condition which had been grown in Washington State. These technologies also have increased the number of choices in the stores. I have encountered citrus imports from Israel, Morocco, South Africa, Chile, and Australia; mangoes are imported from Hawaii and many Caribbean countries and South American countries. There are now other native fruits from all over the world that I had never seen before in our area and they are available in the store in very good condition.

Several companies are doing research to expand controlled atmosphere technology and apply it to other fruits.

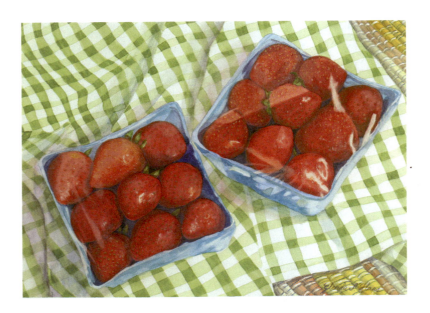

Appendix 2: FRUIT CALENDAR

This calendar is in 3 parts: (1) constitutes the information obtained from experts in the fruit trade, (2) and (3) is the information I have obtained by frequent (at least twice a week) visits to fruit markets. The reader should be aware that every year is different with the vicissitudes of climate and the produce the merchants decide to present at any one time.

This calendar at best will give only an indication of what the reader could expect to find when visiting fruit stores at a particular time of year.

(1) Average availability dates for fruit crops in Northeastern U.S.

Apples – In New Jersey, the fresh apple season starts in mid to late August.

Apple harvest time for individual varieties:

Cameo: Mid October
Cortland: Mid September
Crispin (Mutsu): Early October
Empire: Mid-late September
Fortune: Early October
Fuji: Late October
Ginger Gold*: Late August
Golden Delicious: Late September – early October
Honeycrisp: Early September – Late September
Jonagold: Early October
Macintosh: Early September
Macoun: Late September

Red Delicious: late September
Winesap: Mid-late October

Apricots: Early to late July

Blackberries: August through mid-September

Blueberries: Mid-June to late July

Cherries – Sweet: Late June – Late July
Tart: Early – mid July

Figs (with protection): Late July to early September

Gooseberries: Early July – early August

Nectarines: Late July to late August

Peaches: Mid-July to Mid-September

Pears – Bartlett: Mid-late August
Bosc: Early-mid September
Seckel: Late August – early September

Plums – Japanese: Mid-July to late August
Italian: Late August to mid September

Raspberries: Mid-July to mid-September

Red Currants: Late June – mid July

Strawberries: Late May to late June

The above table was compiled from information kindly supplied by Mark Cole of Demarest Farms, Washington Township, NJ and Glen DePiero of the DePiero Farms, Montvale, NJ.

(2) Fruits with year around availability:

Apples

Avocados

Bananas

Blueberries (Great price fluctuations with the season)

Cantaloupes

Grapes (some types)

Grapefruit
Honeydew melons
Lemons
Limes
Mangoes
Oranges
Papayas
Pears
Pineapples
Plums (some types)
Raspberries
Strawberries
Watermelons

(3) Author's observations in New Jersey fruit stores as to availability.*,**

Chilean cherries
   November 22nd – February 11th

California oranges
   December – April 15th

Florida oranges
   December – April 25th

Most citrus fruits
   January – April

White grapefruit
   January 18th – March 24th

Good Chilean peaches and nectarines
   January 19th

Comice pears
   January 22nd – June 30th

Florida strawberries
> May 17th

New Jersey strawberries
> May 21st – June 30th

California peaches and nectarines
> May 22nd – September 20th

California apricots
> May 13th

Georgia peaches
> May 15th

U.S. cherries
> May 16th - August

New Jersey peaches
> July 9th

New Jersey nectarines
> August 3rd

South African clementines
> August 3rd

Cranberries
> September 28th – January 31st

Fresh figs
> August 15th through October

Prune-plums
> August 20th through September 21st

* *Where only one date is given, it's only of one observation. Usually, the earliest for the year.*

***These dates change somewhat from year to year*

Appendix 3: SUGGESTIONS FOR ON THE SPOT EVALUATION

All Fruits:

All fruits should be examined for appearance, texture and aroma in order not to spend money for inferior produce. Watch out particularly for fruit which has signs of decay or is too unripe.

Apples:

Know what you want to use them for; if for eating fresh, buy those which are available in the orchards at that time or which have not been stored for more than three months after harvest. For eating I especially recommend Golden Delicious and Macoun among the medium hard apples, Fuji, Winesap and Mutsu among the hard, and Cortland among the soft. Look for bruises, other physical damage or wrinkled skin. Never buy an apple that you know has fallen to the ground; bruises will show up later.

Apricots:

Only buy ripe fruit with good aroma and avoid purchasing fruit with any off odor. Do not buy apricots when they are too hard (unless you are planning to cook with them), or too soft. Watch for start of spoilage indicated by brown and sometimes soft spots.

Bananas:

Stem end should be slightly green; no black spots or bruises. Organic bananas, if available, are recommended because at times they have a better flavor. When bananas are totally green, do not buy them as it is much harder to gauge their quality and time when they will be ready for eating.

Cherries:

Check for uniformity, do not purchase when the crate contains soft or rotten fruit or too many cherries with cracks or wrinkled skin. If possible, taste one or two cherries before buying.

Grapes:

Watch for taste, pulpiness and tough skin; should not have brown discolored areas at stem end; if too many grapes have separated from the stems that is a negative. Most people prefer seedless grapes. If at all possible taste one sample grape before buying.

Melons:

Cantaloupe usually ripens in one to four days after purchase. When fruit is aromatic it should be preferred. When there is off or unpleasant odor, do not purchase. Honeydew melons should have a slight give when pressed with the finger; a pleasant aroma is a good indicator for good- for-eating fruit. Honeydew melons, if completely hard and without sweet-aromatic odor can take two to four weeks or more to ripen at room temperature. Occasionally they never ripen to a good flavor, particularly in the off-season when they have been stored for too long. Crenshaw melons: aroma and slight give indicates good eating. Some melons, particularly Cantaloupe, at times have a chemical or perfume taste and odor that cannot be detected from outside the fruit, and is particularly prevalent in late fall.

Nectarines:

Watch for good aroma, and skin that is not leathery. The fruit should show some softness to the touch but not too much.

Oranges:

Look for fruit that is heavy for its size. Color does not affect quality. A wrinkled or loose skin may be a sign indicating that you have a fruit which has been stored for a long time and is undesirable and too dried out, yielding little juice.

Other Citrus Fruits:

Grapefruit: the same criteria as for oranges. This fruit comes with white, pink or red flesh. I personally find the white grapefruit to usually have the best flavor. Clementines, Mandarins and other citrus fruit should be of good color and texture with no special criteria for rejection as long as they have sound appearance. Proportion of weight to size should be high, showing that there has been no drying out of the fruit.

Peaches:

Aroma is most important; should have no wrinkled spots, no damage to the skin, should have some "give" when touched and there should be no deep groove or indentations. Do not buy after mid September as flesh often is mealy and low in flavor. If one peach from a batch is mealy probably most fruits from that batch are of poor quality.

Pears:

Fruit should not be too soft nor have dark areas, brown or black, distinct from the main color of the pear.

Pineapples:

Slightly soft to the touch and some good pineapple aroma at stem end indicate a good fruit, also leaves should not resist too much, when removed by pulling.

Plums:

Only purchase the plums when they are completely ripe but not over-ripe. Must not be dark brown or rotten near the pit (for Italian Plums). It is often best to buy two or three so you can sample them, then decide whether you want to purchase larger amounts. Caution! Some plums have pieces of wood originating from the pit in the flesh and if you do not know this, it could injure you. Black plums should not be bought when unripe; they often rot and ripen simultaneously.

Strawberries:

Aroma and appearance should be the deciding factor for purchase. There must be no moldy odor indicating spoilage or plastic odor from the package. The fruit should have minimum white (not ripe) areas. At times berries from containers tightly packaged in green plastic develop an "artificial" odor and taste.

Dr. Gerhard Haas

Dr. Gerhard Haas, scientist and inventor, grew up in a medical family in Germany where his parents owned and operated a hospital. He left in 1936 to escape Nazism and to study Natural Sciences at Trinity College, Cambridge, England. After university, his first scientific research position was in Cuba. He immigrated to the U.S. in 1943 where his parents had also fled from Germany, and he joined Hoffman la Roche as a senior chemist working with vitamins. He returned to academia for a PhD in microbiology and then followed a successful career in the pharmaceutical and food science industries. He was with General Foods as a microbiologist and enzymologist for 26 years. Over his career he achieved more than 40 patents and 50 publications. (He had applied for his first patent at the age of 14!).

On retiring from General Foods he accepted a research position at the New York Botanical Garden and was adjunct professor in the Biology Department at Lehman College of the City University of New York. In 1992 he transferred his teaching and research to Fairleigh Dickinson University, New Jersey.

Dr. Haas's life in science has spanned six decades—as biochemist, enzymologist and microbiologist, working with some of science's foremost researchers and some of the world's largest pharmaceutical, brewing and food concerns.

This book represents his wish to pass on some of his experience and knowledge of fruit so that the general consumer may enjoy and benefit from the many varieties of fruit from all over the world.

Also from Royal Fireworks Press: *A Scientist's Survival Guide*, by Dr. Gerhard J. Haas. ISBN: 978-0-89824-363-5